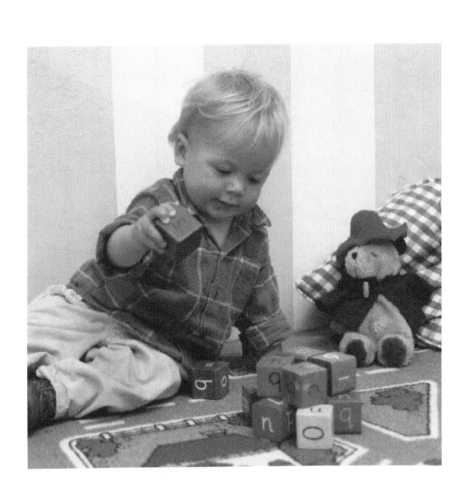

LEADBABIES

How heavy metals are causing our children's autism, ADHD,
learning disabilities, low IQ and behavior problems

Joanna Cerazy M.Ed. and Sandra Cottingham Ph.D.

iUNIVERSE, INC.
NEW YORK   BLOOMINGTON

Lead Babies
How heavy metals are causing our children's autism, ADHD,
learning disabilities, low IQ and behavior problems

iUniverse books may be ordered through booksellers or by contacting:

iUniverse
1663 Liberty Drive
Bloomington, IN 47403
www.iuniverse.com
1-800-Authors (1-800-288-4677)

Because of the dynamic nature of the Internet, any Web addresses or links contained in this book may have changed since publication and may no longer be valid. The views expressed in this work are solely those of the author and do not necessarily reflect the views of the publisher, and the publisher hereby disclaims any responsibility for them.

ISBN: 978-1-4401-8807-7 (sc)
ISBN: 978-1-4401-8806-0 (ebk)

Printed in the United States of America

iUniverse rev. date: 6/1/2010

CONTENTS

ABOUT THE AUTHORS

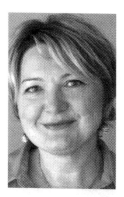

Joanna Cerazy

The book's authors have a long history as teaching colleagues and research partners. They have collaborated on several projects within the field of special education. *Lead Babies* is their first collaborative book.

Joanna Cerazy has a Master's Degree in Educational Leadership with research in special education. She has an extensive background in European and world literature. She has taught both regular and special education in primary, elementary and secondary school contexts. She currently works as a special education consultant. Joanna Cerazy has led and actively participated in several major educational research projects. Recent research includes the skills and knowledge for inclusive education, teacher preparation and special educational policy.

ABOUT THE AUTHORS

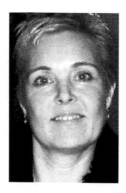

Sandra Cottingham

Sandra Cottingham, M.Sc., Ph.D. has twenty years of classroom experience with regular students and with students with special needs. As a consultant in a large British Columbia school district, Dr. Cottingham works daily with teachers and administrators supporting children with significant cognitive and behavior challenges. Dr. Cottingham's understanding of the issues in special education, her research, and her written work have been recognized by the B.C. Minister of Education. She has been an instructor in the Department of Counseling Psychology and Special Education at the University of British Columbia and a guest presenter for Simon Fraser University. Dr. Cottingham's doctoral dissertation entitled, *Implementing the Mandate of Inclusion, A Model for Moving from Concept to Action* was recently published by Tilburg University, Faculty of Social and Behavioral Sciences, in the Netherlands. Recently, she was named as an Associate of the Taos Institute of New Mexico, USA.

FOREWORD

A nation-wide disregard for warnings about lead due to misinformation and misunderstanding is causing an epidemic of learning and behavior problems in our children. Lead is in the media daily, while growing concern about the global trend of increasing learning and behavior problems in children is at a peak. Fortunately, the future is a hopeful one; the lack of awareness that has allowed a generation of injured children to be born can be replaced with the understanding needed to break the cycle and reverse this needless trend. *Lead Babies* is a book that has the power to initiate profound change.

House paint, gasoline, canned food and tap water: a generation ago, these lead sources changed the world we live in and upped the ante in the gamble that goes with having healthy, thriving children. Despite a recent renewed concern about lead, the lead industry continues to be alive and well with a flourishing demand and steady production. The multiplicity of preventable or removable lead sources that you now invite into your daily routines unintentionally have life-altering consequences.

But there is good news. The cycle of learning disabilities, ADHD, behavior problems and declining IQ, and possibly even autism *can* be broken. As you are shown the tangible links between exposure to lead, the developing brain and children's learning and behavior, you will begin to realize and use the power you have. Each one of us can take small steps to directly and significantly influence our family's future.

Lead sources are easy and inexpensive to identify, reduce and eliminate without radical lifestyle changes. And although damage is irreversible, past lead accumulations from exposure can and *must* be reversed to protect against further, future damage.

For decades, the negative effects on the brain caused by lead have been well understood and documented by neurologists and researchers. Until now, this knowledge has not been presented in practical terms. *Lead Babies* enhances readers' understanding of the costs should they opt for complacency. A small individual effort to reduce and avoid lead will impact a family's quality of life immediately and for generations to come.

This book will change your perceptions and understandings about children's learning, intelligence and behavior today. At very least, you will view the fields of medicine and education through a new lens. Your understanding of people in general will necessarily shift. You will rethink crime. The responsibility of pregnancy will assume new significance. As you reconnect cause with effect, you will have engaged in the first step towards breaking a cycle of lead-caused intellectual disability, the implications of which have the potential to undermine life and society as we know them. At a personal level, your empowerment will shape the legacy you leave in ways that are not only real but profound.

INTRODUCTION

A generation of children struggles to sit still, concentrate, read and understand social cues. Their school programs are modified as they fall behind in school. The impulsiveness that makes them difficult to manage in the classroom becomes a liability in the workplace. These are lead babies, statistics in an epidemic of learning and behaviorally challenged children and young people. Their brains, at key stages of development, primarily in the days, weeks and months following their conception, were permanently damaged by exposure to the dangerous neurotoxin, lead.

There are few toxic substances that have been more studied and more warned about than lead, yet it seems that the information has bypassed most of us.

The next time you sit down for tea, scoop three individual granules of sugar into the palm of your hand. If this were lead, it would be more than enough to permanently damage an infant's brain, whether born or a fetus still growing and forming in the womb. In utero lead exposure in proportions as seemingly insignificant as what you have in your hand inhibits the ability to read, learn, concentrate and behave later on. Accumulated exposure well into adulthood has implications for diminishing IQ and disease that are equally devastating to individuals, families and society. The ripple effect that lead exposure sets into motion has profound and far-reaching implications.

One of the benefits of belonging to the human race is our capacity for change. While we cannot change the brain damage that lead exposure has already rendered permanent, we can make choices and take steps toward breaking the cycle of another generation with learning disabilities, declining intelligence, ADHD, behavior problems and even autism. With a new understanding and an appreciation for lead exposure risk, the cycle of brain-damaged children can be broken. It is ours to break.

CHAPTER 1

LEAD: A CHRONOLOGY

Lead has been man's companion in his journey through the ages. It can be traced back as far as the Bronze Age, with mention of it in the Book of Exodus in the Old Testament of the Bible. It was first discovered in 6500 BC in the mines of Mesopotamia, modern day Turkey. The oldest preserved artifact, a statuette that dates as far back as 3800 BC, can be viewed in the British Museum in London. We have been taking advantage of lead's versatile qualities for thousands of years.

The ancients regarded lead as the father of all metals. Lead was personified as Saturn, the cruel titan who ate his own children. "The very word 'saturnine,' in its most specific meaning, applies to an individual whose temperament has become uniformly gloomy, cynical, and taciturn as the results of lead intoxication."[1]

The rise of the Roman Empire incorporated a widespread use of lead. In analyzing the sequence of events that hastened Rome's demise, we find a list of commonly agreed factors that include Christianity, overindulgence, as well as financial and military problems. However, there was enough lead and documented lead toxicity amongst the elite of Rome to sink a ship. And apparently, to undermine an empire.

Historians pore over examples of the many documented uses of lead. It was used in cosmetics, paint, pharmaceuticals and food. It was prized as a sweetener, added to condiments and used as a preservative. Besides its obvious use in coins, most kitchen cookery and tableware were made of lead-containing pewter. It is how Rome accessed its daily supply of water: through lead pipes. The term *plumbing* comes from the Latin word for lead: *plumbum.* By far, the largest amount of lead used by the Romans was in their extensive aqueducts and water mains. Jack Lewis, writing for the US Environmental Protection Agency, describes what the Romans did and did not know about lead. Ironically, the miscalculation they made about chronic low-level exposure is prevalent today:

> The Romans were aware that lead could cause serious health problems, even madness and death. However, they were so fond of its diverse uses that they minimized the hazards it posed. Romans of yesteryear, like Americans of today, equated limited exposure to lead with limited risk. What they did not realize was that their everyday low-level exposure to the metal rendered them vulnerable to chronic lead poisoning, even while it spared them the full horrors of acute lead poisoning.
>
> The symptoms of acute lead intoxication appeared most vividly among miners who were thrown into unhealthy intimacy with the metal on a daily basis. Romans reserved such debilitating and backbreaking labor for slaves. Some of these unfortunates were forced to spend all of their brief and blighted lives underground, out of sight and out of mind. The unpleasantness of lead mining was further neutralized late in the Empire when the practice was prohibited in Italy and consigned completely to the provinces.
>
> Lead smelting, which had once been commonplace in every Roman city and town, eventually followed

mining operations to the provinces. Italy, the heart of imperial Rome, grew tired of the noxious fumes emanating from lead smelting forges. The obvious damage to the health of smithies and their families was a matter of little or no concern.

Roman aristocrats, who regarded labor of any sort as beneath their dignity, lived oblivious to the human wreckage on which their ruinous diet of lead depended. They would never dream of drinking wine except from a golden cup, but they thought nothing of washing down platters of lead-seasoned food with gallons of lead-adulterated wine. The result, according to many modern scholars, was the death by slow poisoning of the greatest empire the world has ever known.

Symptoms of "plumbism" or lead poisoning were already apparent as early as the first century B.C. Julius Caesar for all his sexual ramblings was unable to beget more than one known offspring. Caesar Augustus, his successor, displayed not only total sterility but also a cold indifference to sex.

The first century A.D. was a time of unbridled gluttony and drunkenness among the ruling oligarchs of Rome. The lead concealed in the food and wine they devoured undoubtedly had a great deal to do with the outbreak of unprecedented epidemics of saturnine gout and sterility among aristocratic males and the alarming rate of infertility and stillbirths among aristocratic women.

Still more alarming was the conspicuous pattern of mental incompetence that came to be synonymous with the Roman elite. This creeping cretinism manifested itself most frighteningly in such clearly degenerate emperors as Caligula, Nero, and Commodus. It is said that Nero wore a breastplate of lead, ostensibly to strengthen his voice, as he fiddled and sang while Rome burned. Domitian, the last of the Flavian emperors, actually had a fountain installed in his palace from which he could drink a never-ending stream of leaded wine.[2]

On the heels of the Roman Empire came the Middle Ages, when only some of the lessons that had been learned about lead would be passed on; other bad decisions involving lead were destined to be repeated. Lead's lethal properties were employed in sinister plots to quietly eliminate "problem" individuals. Alchemists believed lead could play a role in generating much sought after gold from other baser metals. Most noteworthy though, was lead's predominance as a material in guns and weaponry, and the mass production of lead-based ammunition ensued.

Many attempts were made to prevent lead poisoning. As early as A.D. 802, Charlemagne is reputed to have prohibited the use of lead in wine. In later ages, the practice of adulterating wine with lead became so widespread that it had to be officially banned by the Imperial Law of 1498. Edict or not, the practice continued.[3]

Throughout the ages, the extensive use of lead in various cooking utensils for food and wine preparation caused recurring outbreaks of lead poisoning. These outbreaks, almost always traced to lead-containing food or drink, were referred to as colic. There was the colic of Poitou caused by wine in France, the colic of Devonshire linked to cider in England, the *entrapado* of Spain caused by lead-containing cooking vessels, and the so called dry bellyache caused by rum and other drinks experienced by the colonial Americans.[4] Lead colic endemics caused by the lead contained in alcoholic beverages and lead poisoning caused by lead-adulterated foods were certainly not a rarity. On the contrary, they were common indispositions in colonial America and other countries.

One technological advance invited another and change was constant. Whereas the Romans had used lead as a sweetener, the King of England discovered his own contemporary alternative: sugar. First introduced to Great Britain in the 1300s, it was a rare and exotic treat reserved for the occasional indulgence of the privileged and wealthy. King Henry VIII had considerable means, reach and appetite. Joined by the members of his court, he indulged with a vengeance. Consequently, they experienced such sugar-induced tooth decay that the profession of dentistry literally was sprung into existence. Lead was initially used to fill dental caries in Henry's time; however, the use of mercury became prevalent in later centuries.

New uses for lead were discovered during the Industrial Revolution of the mid-eighteenth century. As the first colonies established themselves in the New World, the same type of mines that centuries before had been relegated to the provinces of Italy began to be established in the Virginias. "By 1621 the metal was being mined and forged in Virginia. The low melting temperature of lead made it highly malleable, even at the most primitive forges. Furthermore, lead's resistance to corrosion greatly enhanced its strength and durability. Technological progress in the American colonies and the American republic was to owe a great deal to this useful and abundant metal."[5] Among other uses, lead began to be utilized in the manufacture of ammunition and glassware and it found its way into the printing process.

By the early nineteenth century, occupational lead exposure played an important role in the unfolding drama of lead's harm. Occupational exposure brought the rapid realization that lead not only affected the individuals involved directly in a given lead industry but also their spouses and children. More and more cases of sterility, miscarriage, stillbirth and premature delivery were reported (see chapter 8).

Children of parents who worked with lead were often born with congenital disabilities. Their chances of survival after being born were very slim compared to other infants. Children who did survive often suffered from conditions such as delayed development, macrocephaly (enlarged head) and convulsive seizures. A physician of the time described children who were exposed to lead: they "do not grow up into capable men and women like other children, but they are handicapped in their start in life and that subsequently many of them exhibit signs of mental as well as physical deterioration."[6] In a novel, *The Uncommercial Traveler*, Charles Dickens describes the horrible effects of occupational lead poisoning in women in the mid-nineteenth century:

> 'The lead, sur. Sure 'tis the lead-mills, where the women gets took on at eighteen-pence a day, sur, when they makes application early enough, and is lucky and wanted; and 'tis lead-pisoned she is, sur, and some of them gets lead-pisoned soon, and some of them gets

> lead-pisoned later, and some, but not many, niver; and
> 'tis all according to the constitooshun, sur, and some
> constitooshuns is strong, and some is weak; and her
> constitooshun is lead-pisoned, bad as can be, sur; and
> her brain is coming out at her ear, and it hurts her
> dreadful; and that's what it is, and niver no more, and
> niver no less, sur.'[7]

Eventually, once labor laws were passed to address growing concerns, women were banned from jobs that involved significant lead exposure. In light of such laws, some companies began to bar women from all jobs that had any exposure to lead unless the women provided a medical note that they were already infertile. Consequently, some women felt they had no choice but to get sterilized in order to remain employed. Many perceived this as the solution to the problem of lead poisoning itself. In hindsight, it shows the lack of understanding at that time of lead's toxic effect on the fertility of both women and men.

The mystery of the famous Franklin Expedition to the Northwest Passage in the mid-1840s was for many years unsolved. It was May 19, 1845 when the two ships, the HMS *Terror* and the HMS *Erebus,* set sail from Europe. Both ships were fully stocked with tins of food to last up to three years. The ships' unexplained disappearance in the second year of the voyage was probed extensively over the next decade with numerous expeditions setting out after them. Eventually, when the evidence was collected and examined, a consensus emerged. The demise of the crew was the result of a number of factors, not the least of which was a series of uncharacteristically poor decisions. The forensic evidence collected from the frozen bodies of the men, coupled with the remnant tins that had supplied their food throughout the journey, revealed that the underlying cause in the death of the captain and the 125 men aboard was lead poisoning from the lead solder used to seal the tin cans. This explained not only their deaths but the string of poor decisions that contributed to the catastrophe.[8]

In 1892, the first reports of the harm caused by leaded paint to children came from Australia. At first, ten cases of lead palsy were reported, its cause a complete mystery. It took over a decade for the involved physicians to discover and document that the causes of these children's conditions came from their own homes, more specifically from the paint on the railings and walls. Warnings emerged that lead was also contained in house dust and that children's hand-to-mouth activities increase the amount of lead children consume.[9]

This admonition, unfortunately for all of us, was promptly forgotten and lead continued to silently interfere with the wellbeing of millions of future children. Despite Australia's obvious need to prohibit the use of lead in paint, the allowable lead limit was merely set at 0.1 percent for house paint. It was not until 1997 that lead was banned in paint.

Despite earlier claims that this mystery disease was exclusive to the Australian continent, incidents of lead poisoning began to be reported two decades later in North America. By the early 1920s, the ill effects of lead were well understood and documented. Ruddock, for example, in 1924, indicated food coloring, food containers and medicinal ointment as possible sources of lead.[10] Eighty-nine cases of lead poisoning, eleven of which were fatal, were soon reported from Boston. Incidents of lead poisoning and death were becoming more and more common. At that time, the most frequent sources of lead were described as paint coming from woodwork, furniture and toys.[11] Today, almost a century later, lead is still used in our children's bibs, cribs and toys.

The greatest increase in human exposure to lead began when, despite existing warnings of its potential harmful effects, lead was incorporated into gasoline as an anti-knock agent in the 1920s. The lead compound, tetraethyl lead, eventually known simply as ethyl, was added to petroleum to boost the octane rating. Not coincidentally, its fantastic success became the "boost" the automobile industry needed. Beginning in 1922, approximately a quarter-million tons of lead compounds entered the atmosphere each year.

As early as 1924, during tests on ethyl, several workers suddenly became violently ill, delirious and died of acute lead poisoning. Over time, a growing number of workers met the same fate although it would be fifty more years before a ban would be put in place.

In the 1930s and 1940s, many children were affected by lead's toxicity. In the early 1930s several large American cities reported mass lead poisoning among poor families. The source for these outbreaks, later called the *Depression Disease*, turned out to be fumes from the battery casings these families used for fuel in cold weather. As a result of this and other exposures, many children died and many remained seriously disabled. Even the children who were "cured" were later found to do poorly at school. Many children showed signs of sensorimotor deficits and behavior problems such as impulsivity and short attention span. It would take the scientific community another thirty years to produce controlled investigations that documented the debilitating effects of low-level lead exposure.

Between 1950 and 1960, lead poisoning became commonplace amongst children. Mortality associated with it was extremely high. Cases upon cases were uncovered and reported: 611 cases with forty-eight deaths reported in Baltimore; 143 cases with thirty-nine deaths reported in New York City; 223 cases with forty-one deaths reported in Philadelphia; and 429 cases with sixty-seven deaths reported in Chicago.[12] Notably, lead poisoning occurred almost exclusively in children one to six years of age with children newborn to three years of age at the greatest risk. The highest incidence was reported for ethnic minorities and the economically disadvantaged.

This shocking data on lead-induced damage to children had a minimal effect on health workers at the time and on society at large. The first national mass-screening program started in Chicago did not begin until 1966. Quickly followed by similar programs in other US cities, these initiatives revealed that lead poisoning was more widespread than was initially reputed. Data obtained from screening programs revealed that lead poisoning was not exclusive to the so-called "lead belts" of the poor. Attention was drawn to thousands of asymptomatic children with unduly elevated levels of blood-lead. Simultaneously, reports of similar problems were beginning to emerge from other countries.

These events highlighted several key facts about lead's toxicity. Children's extreme vulnerability to lead became evident, as did lead's harmful effects on the central nervous system. It was clear that low, sub-clinical blood-lead levels previously believed to be safe were causing harm. Moreover, a disease that had been considered an affliction of the poor and uneducated became recognized as a national and worldwide problem.

Cases of lead poisoning were now everywhere. In the 1960s, twenty-three cases were treated in Ontario, Canada. A study from Chile revealed that out of seventy-six sand workers' children, sixty had blood-lead levels exceeding thirty micrograms per deciliter, a startlingly high amount considering that currently the US Centers for Disease Control and Prevention considers ten micrograms the "level of concern" for lead in the bloodstream. This amount is even more alarming in light of new evidence that indicates that "the only *safe* level of lead exposure for children and pregnant women is no exposure."[13]

In Sydney, Australia, ninety cases of children with high blood-lead levels were reported. Twenty-two cases were diagnosed in Germany. In England and Wales, ninety-nine children under the age of five died from lead exposure. Reports were coming from around the world; Auckland, New Zealand, Kuwait, Sri Lanka, Belgium and Italy, with unknown numbers of cases unreported and untreated.

Faced with irrefutable data, the US Surgeon General issued a statement that emphasized the importance of childhood prevention of lead poisoning. A year later, Congress became involved and the 1971 Lead-Based Paint Poisoning Prevention Act ensued. According to this new Act, the lead content of paint used for residential structures, furniture, eating utensils and toys was set as no more than 0.06 percent.

The process of adjusting "acceptable" blood-lead levels had begun back in the 1960s. It was first lowered from eighty micrograms per deciliter to sixty micrograms per deciliter. Forty micrograms per deciliter was deemed to be a desirable level in 1971. In 1975, the US Centers for Disease Control lowered it again, this time to thirty micrograms per deciliter. A decade later, this level was adjusted again to twenty-five micrograms per deciliter. And subsequently, in 1991 it was decreased to ten micrograms per deciliter, where it remains.

The World Health Organization followed in 1995. In light of data showing that levels lower than ten micrograms per deciliter cause cognitive deficits in children, who then exhibit deficits in working memory and behavioral flexibility,[14] the argument persists that there is no safe blood-lead level and the current maximum value needs to be reduced further.

In the 1980s, dietary lead consumption came under scrutiny. Lead content in canned baby food, evaporated milk and other food staples was proven to be unacceptably high. In 1991, the US Food and Drug Administration announced a program to reduce wine-originating consumer exposure to lead and set limits on maximum amounts of lead allowable in food. Leaded solder was abandoned by the American food industry: regrettably, it may still be used in other countries.

There is an unfortunate parallel between the announcements that leaded gasoline and paint containing lead were to end. The announced retraction and subsequent celebration conveyed a message that lead was gone and the world was now safe, when nothing could be further from the truth. What happened instead is that lead fell from people's radar, and the growing understanding of the harmful effects of lead that initiated the need to stop its use gave way to a generation of consumers (and parents-to-be) with neither fear nor knowledge. There was a deadly wrong assumption that the lead problem had been taken care of, and a new generation emerged with no idea that there had ever been a problem in the first place.

Lead in gasoline for on-road vehicles was first banned in Canada in 1990. America followed with its Clean Air Act in 1996. With the exception of some developing countries, the use of lead in fuels for on-road vehicles was subsequently banned in most places in the world. Leaded gasoline is still standard for off-road use, used extensively in farm equipment, marine engines and race cars. For those who were under the impression that lead in fuels was a thing of the past—most propeller-driven airplanes continue to use leaded gas.

Paint has remained a major contaminator and lead exposure source. The lead compound in paint was used as pigment, as well as to speed the drying process, increase durability, and resist moisture that eventually would cause erosion. While the use of lead in interior paint was either banned or restricted in many countries during the early decades of the twentieth century, no such regulations were established in the United States. To the contrary, in the 1920s, the Lead Industries Association undertook a campaign promoting the use of lead in paint. The Dutch Boy logo became a familiar symbol and a household name of the twentieth century. The claims made by the lead industry to promote its products are outrageous by today's standards.

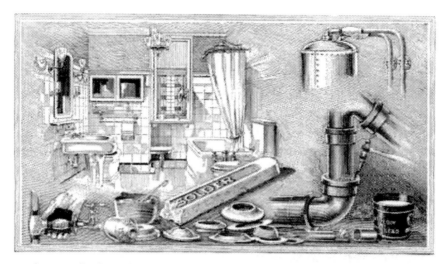

Lead helps to guard your health

YOU wouldn't live today in a house without an adequate plumbing system. For without modern plumbing, sickness might endanger your life.

Lead concealed in the walls and under the floors of many modern buildings helps to give the best sanitation.

Lead pipe centuries old

Lead, therefore, is contributing to the health, comfort, and convenience of people today as it did when Rome was a center of civilization. Lead water and drainage pipes more than 1800 years old have been found in exactly the condition they were in when laid.

In some cities today the law specifies that lead pipe alone may be used to bring water from street mains into the building.

In drainage systems are lead traps made of lead pipe bent into the shape of the letter S, so that a little water will stay in the bend and prevent gases which collect in the pipe from getting out through the house.

The malleability of lead also makes it easy to change the direction of any pipe through the use of lead bends.

Joining the pipes

A plumber easily "wipes" a joint or repairs a pipe leak with lead and tin solder. Because this alloy melts at the low temperature of 358 degrees it can be applied without melting the lead pipe, which melts at 620 degrees.

Lead is also pressed into the flanges of pipe-joints to make them absolutely tight. Pipe threads are painted with white-lead or red-lead to make a tight connection. Where vibration or movement of pipes may loosen a poured joint, lead wool is used; lead shredded into threads is packed into the joint in a dense, compact mass.

Rubber gaskets and ball washers containing lead prevent leaking at joints and faucets.

Lead is used to beautify the modern bathroom. Red-lead and litharge, both lead oxides, are important ingredients in making the glossy white enamel covering the iron bodies of tub and basin and the glazed tile walls.

Lead in paint

While lead is invaluable in assuring comfort and proper sanitation, its best-known and most widespread use is as white-lead in paint. Such materials as wood would soon deteriorate unless protected with paint. And the paints that give the most thorough protection against the weather are based on white-lead.

The loss of invested capital through failure to protect the surface of property adequately has led property owners to paint frequently and well. As days and months go by, more and more of them are learning the wisdom of the phrase, "Save the surface and you save all." And they are using white-lead paint to prolong the lives of their houses.

Look for the Dutch Boy

NATIONAL LEAD COMPANY makes white-lead and sells it mixed with pure linseed oil, under the name and trade-mark of Dutch Boy white-lead. The figure of the Dutch Boy is reproduced on every keg and is a guarantee of exceptional purity.

Dutch Boy products also include red-lead, linseed oil, flatting oil, babbitt metals and solder.

More about lead

If you use lead, or think you might use it in any form, write to us for specific information.

NATIONAL LEAD COMPANY

New York, 111 Broadway; Boston, 131 State St.; Buffalo, 116 Oak St.; Chicago, 900 West 18th St.; Cincinnati, 659 Freeman Ave.; Cleveland, 820 West Superior Ave.; St. Louis, 722 Chestnut St.; San Francisco, 485 California St.; Pittsburgh, National Lead & Oil Co. of Pa., 316 Fourth Ave.; Philadelphia, John T. Lewis & Bros. Co., 437 Chestnut St.

In an attempt to secure future markets, the US lead industry turned to children as prime targets. Paint distributors advised store owners not to forget the children. Several paint books encouraging the use of lead paint were produced for children. One of them, *A Paint Book for Girls and Boys*, depicted the Dutch Boy, bucket and brush in hand, looking at the "lead family"—lead soldiers, shoe soles, light bulbs, etc. Another paint book showing the Dutch Boy using lead paint to paint walls and furniture suggested that by doing so "Dutch Boy Conquers Old Man Gloom:"

The girl and boy felt blue
Their toys were old and shabby too,
They couldn't play in such a place,
The room was really a disgrace.

The famous Dutch Boy Lead of mine
Can make this playroom fairly shine
Let's start our painting right away
You'll find the work is only play.[15]

Cater
To The Children

Do you make it a point in your store to show courtesy to your youthful customers? Do you give them the same consideration and attention that you do the older folks, or do you brush them aside as of less importance?

Have you stopped to think that the children of today are the grown-ups of tomorrow and that a child is particularly quick to remember a kindness and slow to forget a slight or an injustice?

A busy parent sends a child —perhaps a shy little girl— to make a purchase. If there is a choice of stores, the child naturally makes a practice of going where she is made to feel welcome and where she is waited on promptly. She wins approval for doing her errand quickly and it takes less time from her own interests.

This is one of the seemingly small matters which many successful merchants consider worth attention.

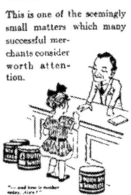

12

Despite the fact that in 1978 the limit of lead in interior paint was lowered to 0.06 percent, lead paint still abounds in older houses where it was originally applied. In 1992, the Lead-Based Paint Hazard Reduction Act in the United States known as Title X (Title Ten) provided law regulating lead paint. One of its key clauses is the requirement to disclose any lead hazards known at the time of sale or lease of a home that was built before 1978. Removing lead-containing paint can cost tens of thousands of dollars per single dwelling. According to a 2000 US Environmental Protection Agency report, it would cost fifty-eight billion dollars to remove leaded paint across the United States.

The story of industrial paint presents an even grimmer picture. Lead is still allowed in paint used to cover industrial structures such as bridges and machinery. Lead-containing paint is favored due to its ability to expand and contract with the metal surface without cracking, as well as its resistance to corrosion. Even if leaded paint for industrial use were outlawed today, we would still be exposed to it for years to come as it coats our bridges and numerous other metal structures. In the United States alone there are over 90,000 bridges coated with leaded paint. On occasion, whole communities have had to be relocated while older lead-containing paint-covered structures were renovated.

Human activities have caused such widespread lead contamination in the planet's water cycle and food chain that our lead intake is now one hundred times that of our prehistoric ancestors.

In the year 2000, the US Centers for Disease Control and Prevention estimated that in the United States, there were still 454,000 children with blood-lead concentration greater than ten micrograms per deciliter, and in 2005 it was estimated that more than 300,000 children less than six years of age had blood-lead levels over ten micrograms per deciliter. The numbers may seem encouraging; however, the US Centers for Disease Control and Prevention's focus on these high thresholds of blood-lead levels does not reflect two of the most important factors in lead exposure that are now before us. Cumulative exposure and accumulation of lead in bones and brain tissue are not reflected in the snapshot that blood-lead levels provide. Also, children with far lower blood-lead levels than those counted in the statistics all have a degree of irreversible central nervous system impairment.

Lead exposure, fully understood and easily preventable but nevertheless allowed to degrade generation after generation, is one of the greatest ironies of the human experience. The next generation desperately needs to be the last in the cycle of ignoring lead, a force that is shaping not only individual lives, but the quality of life shared by whole communities. Grasping the intensity of lead's assault on human potential has been a critical first step in empowering readers. But what great news to discover that avoiding lead is as easy as having a plan and applying the knowledge of where to be on the lookout. It is neither difficult nor expensive. While the implications of acting have far-reaching impact at a societal level, tackling the lead issue is personally relevant and beneficial. It must happen immediately. Fortunately, we act when something concerns those about whom we deeply care.

NOTES

CHAPTER 2

LEAD BABIES:
FROM CONCEPTION TO BIRTH

The Millers' Good News

When Sandy Miller received the call from her family doctor confirming her test results, it was hard to catch up to the reality of it all. Since they had uprooted five years ago from the small prairie town just thirty miles from where Sandy had been born and raised, she and her husband Craig had been trying to conceive. She could not be happier that her intuition had been correct. They were expecting their first child.

Sandy had heard the phone ringing from the garden where she had been planting a row of small shrubs across the front of the house. She had run inside, kicking her boots off in the hallway and hurrying to the kitchen just in time and out of breath. Her immediate reaction was to call Craig, but as she retrieved her boots and then returned to the garden outside with the portable phone in hand, she had decided to savor the news and tell him in person when he got home. She had Fridays off from the gallery where she worked as an art appraiser, and

Craig, a supervisor at a nearby oil refinery, would end his day earlier than later knowing she was at home. Trying to contain herself, she grabbed the last of the bag of bone meal, poured it into the awaiting hole with a cloud of dust, and set the root ball of a small Rhododendron into the hole. After adjusting the shrub several times, she backfilled the hole with her hands. The loose dirt was cool and damp under the shade of the eaves. She was lost in thought with plans of a long dreamed about nursery as she smoothed the soil around each of the plants, and wiped her hands off on her jeans. She stood back to admire the finished effect.

The Miller house had been a massive undertaking. They had bought the house just a year after getting married. It was modest, and needed fixing up, but mostly, it had met their criteria of having character and being in their price range. The inside renovations had taken up the last four and a half years, and now finally, the outside had been power-washed and repainted with a palette of heritage colors in keeping with a local community restoration plan. Theirs was a dark earth tone with cream trim and black window sashes. The original house construction was considered Craftsman style dating back to 1925. The renovations couldn't have wrapped up at a better time, Sandy reflected. And then her thoughts returned to the nursery that she was letting herself fully imagine for the first time in several years. She couldn't resist the urge to go right inside and upstairs, and to stand in the unfinished room, presently relegated to storage. She was still standing in amongst the boxes and spare furniture when Craig appeared in the doorway wondering what was up.

That had been three months ago. Now Sandy, obviously pregnant, leaned against a stepladder and sipped herbal tea from her favorite handmade ceramic mug. This was the one room that they had not repainted with the rest of the house. A leak from before they had replaced the roof had done some surface damage to one of the walls, so there had been some significant patching and loose paint removal that had to be done before the new paint was applied. There was a missing window casing that was impossible to match, so the moldings came off and a new set, reminiscent of the old style, went up in their place. The old ones were cut up into kindling and tossed on the woodpile for colder months ahead.

In the basement, a set of nursery furniture had been stripped back to bare wood and sat ready for a new finish. It had been in Craig's family since he was born. Sandy was happy to inherit the set, but had one room design in mind for a boy and a different design for a girl. Until she could find out the sex of her baby, she would be undecided as to whether to stain and keep the rustic wood look for a boy's room, or paint it to go with her plans for a girl's décor. Time, and an ultrasound, would tell.

Sandy was feeling good. She was getting lots of rest, eating well and drinking lots of milk. She was also drinking plenty of water, avoiding caffeine and staying clear of anywhere where there was second-hand smoke. Her plan to continue to work at the gallery for as long as she could was so far not a problem.

As the pregnancy progressed, summer gave way to fall and the start of Sandy's third trimester was marked by the Thanksgiving Day weekend. She insisted on hosting the dinner and cooking the turkey. In the back of Sandy's mind, she could also use the occasion to unveil the finished nursery.

The wood finish on the crib and matching dresser and change table made an obvious statement that, until the room reveal, had been a secret. Craig had spent September repairing a number of broken or missing panes in a small stained glass window that had been removed from the room that was now assigned as the nursery. It took a bit of a research and then some fiddling to fit things fully back together, but thankfully his monopolization of the dining room table had been end-dated by the commitment of Thanksgiving dinner. But the window was stunning and made the finished nursery a showpiece. It was complete with a toy train from Craig's childhood that hadn't been unpacked for probably twenty-five years. They had set it up on the floor of the nursery, and then the two of them had played with it for several hours.

The day before the dinner, Sandy had polished the silver cutlery and serving pieces. Once the turkey was in the oven, she had set the table with their best crystal and a set of china that came out only for special occasions. Sandy had Craig light the first fire of the year in the living room fireplace. She sat in a large chair with her feet on the ottoman as he stacked the kindling and wedged some loosely scrunched balls of newspaper under the grate. On the hearth, Sandy had left a bag jammed with the wrapping paper from a baby shower that her coworkers had thrown her that week, and she reminded Craig to burn it. In minutes the fire was devouring both the paper and the kindling and she could feel the heat radiating towards her.

The crowd for dinner represented both sides of the family, and there was enough discussion about baby names and what so-and-so was like as a baby to endure multiple shifts in the kitchen before and after dinner. When the meal was done and the table needed to be cleared, she was banished to the living room to put her feet up and relax. Someone arrived with her wine goblet, which had been filled with unsweetened grapefruit juice. She sipped it increasingly slowly as it took on the temperature of the room. She imagined how different Thanksgiving was going to look next year.

When Thomas Oliver wrote of the ability of lead to cross the placenta from mother to fetus, it was not difficult to prove since high levels of lead were found in stillborn infants. The year was 1891.

In 2008, more than a century later, expectant mothers are less aware than ever. They seem unaware, unconcerned, or at least unconvinced about the brain damage lead causes, and in consideration of how much information is available, oblivious to its sources. Sandy Miller and her husband, Craig, are typical parents-to-be who are committed to creating a healthy baby and providing for its needs. Yet they unmindfully expose themselves and their unborn child to needless risk, a scenario that repeats itself across the world in real life every day. The detrimental effects of lead do not occur only in other countries, nor are they limited to those who live in poverty. Meanwhile, in utero lead exposure subjects a fetus to potential harm at the most critical and precarious time in a human's life.

The risk of lead exposure to the unborn child is twofold. The ongoing, immediate exposure to the fetus is the most obvious. This is the day in, day out, toxic load that a pregnant mother comes in contact with, depending on where she lives, where she works, what she eats, and who and what she comes in contact with on any given day. A typical pregnant mother is vigilant, at least in avoiding exposure to those things that she is aware she is being exposed to. For instance, quitting smoking, avoiding alcohol or caffeine, and being careful not to use toxic cleaning chemicals are part of pregnancy for most expectant mothers.

A second consideration with regard to lead exposure and the safety of the unborn child is linked to a woman's own lifelong accumulation of lead, sometimes a more significant factor in the amount of lead her unborn child is exposed to during a pregnancy. Blood-lead levels tell us about recent exposure and certainly pose a serious hazard to an unborn child who has no barrier of protection. While an excellent resource for determining how safe a person's environment is right now, blood-lead levels do not speak to the full risk that the unborn child faces. What is equally critical is how much lead a mother has accumulated in her bones and tissue over the course of her lifetime. For some, it is a stunning realization that twenty or thirty years of lead exposure can come to bear on an unborn child over the relatively short duration of a pregnancy. So while the day-to-day exposure of a woman who is pregnant is hugely important, it is only one piece of a larger picture. The lead we are talking about may have come from our own mothers before we were born, but for certain it is a toxicological archive of every day since. Seemingly insignificant exposure levels collect up in bone and brain tissue, much of it remnant from a time when gasoline and paint were all full of lead.

Bone lead accumulation is a very significant element in unborn children's neurological development and ultimately their potential. Before examining the possibilities and options for how to reduce past accumulations and find and eliminate existing sources, it is critical that we connect lead with the disabilities it causes by creating a concrete understanding of how the brain develops. We need to fully appreciate the brain's susceptibility to lead before we can be truly aware of what is needed to protect it. Rather than think of the unborn baby as an abstract concept, or project onto it, an image of an intact fully grown baby, we need to visualize what it really is and what is happening week by week throughout a pregnancy. Only then will the notion of lead fumes from wrapping paper tossed carelessly into an open fireplace, or the decision to polish the silver, become meaningfully connected with a child's struggle to cut paper with scissors, or color inside the lines when his classmates have mastered it easily.

A Chronology of Vulnerability: The First Trimester

How exactly does the human nervous system develop? How soon after fertilization of the egg occurs does the central nervous system begin to form? These are fundamentally important questions to answer in order to have an appreciation and understanding of brain dysfunction if a learning disability, autism, or something as seemingly subjective as a behavior problem, or ADHD occurs.

At Conception

The answer to the question of when development begins is that cell division happens so immediately following fertilization, that within mere hours, distinct areas of the embryo can be identified. This is important information, since each area develops into different parts of the body, organs, etc. It is profound to realize that the foundation for life becomes so highly organized so quickly. It is virtually immediate. By seven weeks, the rate of neuron formation is thousands per minute. By the end of gestation, the completed process of neuron production will have yielded a total of ten billion of them.

Imagine that this complex sequence is a ballet performance and that the developing brain is the stage. Every few moments, a group of dancers splits off and migrates to a different part of the stage. As new groups appear seemingly from out of nowhere, evolving and changing, timing and position are everything; precision is imperative. Someone or something wandering in from the wings unanticipated or unplanned could throw an entire sequence off, if not throw the whole performance into a chaotic response. It is unpredictable what will happen. Whether a dancer misses a step and carries on, trips and falls or becomes lost and confused in the middle of the stage depends on the exact timing of the unplanned guest, their point of entry, and other factors.

Everything in the developing embryo has a specific job to be carried out in a certain way at a certain time. To throw off mechanisms which regulate the intricate processes of proliferation, migration, morphogenesis or differentiation adds significant risk to an already precarious process. As any number of toxic substances enter the dance, the likelihood that development will be impacted and a child's perceptual facility, sensory processing ability or intellectual potential will be compromised, increases.

Week Three

By the seventeenth day of development, the embryo has changed shape, remotely hinting at what its future baby form will one day be. This flattened elongated shape develops a bit of a bulge on the side that faces away from the uterus wall. This bulging is the neuron plate, what will evolve to become the central nervous system. When this bulging is complete, it begins to push back into itself, creating a hollow cavity, not unlike the way the finger of a glove can be pushed back inside itself. Eventually the edges come together forming a tube shape. This is known as the neural tube. The cells making up this neural tube become the neurons that make up the central nervous system. This is the very foundation for the development of the healthy brain; a critical time to avoid exposure to lead.

Week Four

By the time one month has passed following conception, the neural tube has closed itself at both extremities. The cells on the outside of the tube will eventually form every other part of the human body. Those on the inside will become the central nervous system. At three to four weeks, the embryo looks like a pea pod, with three distinct, connected cavities for peas. A cross-section view shows the first stages of what will become the spinal cord, and the three pea-like ventricles of the encephalon, or what we know as the brain.

Week Five

Two of these three ventricles, the forebrain and the hindbrain, each split again by five weeks, and essentially the structural groundwork for the central nervous system has been laid. No more subdivisions are scheduled to occur between now and full maturation of the brain. This forebrain split happens laterally into an anterior and posterior cavity. These are the earlier stages of the right and left cerebral hemispheres of the brain, parts most of us are familiar with. This is a busy week in the development of a brain, as the forebrain split also gives rise to structures that will evolve into the retina and the optic nerve. The hindbrain will eventually control respiratory, digestive, circulatory and fine motor processes. The midbrain will develop into the command center for basic auditory and visual processing.

Week Twelve

As each of the compartments develops, the cavities begin a process of segmentation resulting in a domino effect of brain regions beginning to form. The first version of the cortex appears, followed by the limbic areas. And then, from twelve weeks to seven months, the main portion of the pregnancy, the details fill in.

The cerebral cortex evolves into three vital components. The visual cortex is responsible for high level visual processing. The temporal cortex is responsible for auditory and visual processing, as well as receptive language function. The parietal cortex is responsible for sensory integration and visual-motor processing.

The frontal cortex, responsible for high-level cognition, motor control and expressive language, also begins to form. This cortical development is established prenatally; however, it continues its evolution well into the adolescent years. Other brain components which develop simultaneously at this phase are the basal ganglia, hippocampal formation, amygdala and olfactory bulb, the thalamus and surrounding nuclei, hypothalamus, retina and optic nerve, the pons, the cerebellum and the medulla.

We know that toxic exposure during the first trimester of pregnancy interferes with the migration and organization of brain cells and that any insult at this stage of development affects future brain development stages. Where it was previously supposed that with so little of a human formed little damage could be done, the reverse has been discovered to be true. A foundation with damage will not support what is built on top of it.

The Second Trimester

The second trimester is the time typically associated with the development of fingers, toes and organs. Yet, it is important to recognize that the development of the central nervous system is still not complete. There are poignant examples that demonstrate what an unwelcome and dangerous time it is for lead or other toxins to reach the fetus. While some damage is hidden within the unfinished brain, other is startlingly obvious at birth.

Depending on your age as a reader, you may be familiar with the impact of Thalidomide. This was a drug prescribed to expectant mothers in the late 1950s and early 1960s to combat morning sickness. Over a six-year period, ten thousand children of mothers who were given Thalidomide were born with malformed or missing limbs.

Rubella, commonly known as the German measles, causes defects in the unborn child's heart as it passes from an infected mother through the placenta to the fetus. Prenatal alcohol consumption can cause facial abnormalities and diminished birth weight. The use of retinoids in products to treat acne in an expectant mother causes malformations of the skull and facial region in the unborn child.

In addition to the physical damage caused by these toxic agents, all of them also cause central nervous system damage. The physical changes suggest an alarming amount of damage, and yet the central nervous system is the most vulnerable in the unborn child. It is damage to the central nervous system that creates significant negative impact on an individual's potential for learning and behavior. While the damage caused by lead (a brain with compromised intellect, sensory processing, ability for self-control, modulation of emotion, or prediction of outcomes) is less obvious than the examples of physical congenital defects that we can see and touch, it is nonetheless real, enduring and occurs at far lower levels of toxin exposure than what it takes to change the development of a limb or an ear.

The Third Trimester

During the third trimester, neurotoxic insults severely affect the hippocampus. This is the part of the brain that is primarily responsible for functions related to learning, memory and emotion allowing social and moral values to develop. Lead toxicity at any stage of hippocampal development interferes with this aspect of behavioral development.

The prefrontal cortex, also vulnerable in the third trimester, continues under development right into the adolescent years. Aggression and impulse control are shaped by this frontal lobe.

These facts may provide insight to those who have values and a well-established moral compass and lack empathy and tolerance for those who do not. What they perceive as bad genes, bad parenting or just bad behavior may in many cases be a direct result of damage to the brain caused by early, ongoing or cumulative exposure to the neurotoxin lead. Certainly, as chapter six will explore, evidence of high levels of lead accumulation in bone and tissue correlates closely with delinquency and those in our North American prisons.

CRITICAL PERIODS IN HUMAN DEVELOPMENT

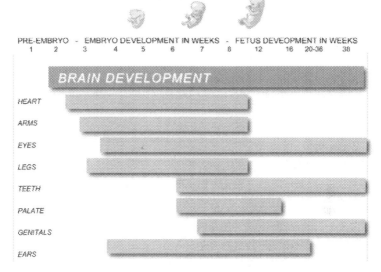

Adapted from *Stages of Developing Fetus*, Minnesota Department of Health, 1999.

Where does lead come from?

In the world of an expectant mother, environmental lead is everywhere and avoidance is simply not as straightforward as choosing the nonsmoking section of a restaurant, declining a glass of wine, or using gentler cleaning agents. The question of where lead comes from and how it enters the human system takes on a new importance in the wake of making a connection between lead exposure and human brain development. A look back at the scenario of Sandy Miller allows us to make vital connections between everyday activities that we all take part in, sources of lead and the vulnerability of the intricate brain development sequence in the unborn child.

First, you will recall the Millers' struggle to conceive. Both Sandy and her husband, Craig, work in settings where lead exposure would be daily and, equally as important, where they would bring home lead particles on their clothes and in their hair. Craig's work at the refinery puts him in close proximity with ongoing exposure to a lead source, leaving him at risk for a lowered sperm count and for producing sperm associated with birth defects, mental retardation and increased miscarriage. Sandy is also in close proximity to art objects and paintings that date from a time when lead was not regulated and was used extensively in artists' supplies.

The bone meal that Sandy was using in the garden contains lead and the cloud of dust formed while dumping out the bag created a scenario where airborne lead particles were likely ingested. The soil that she touched was not only contaminated by years of car exhaust from their busy street but also heavily tainted by the recent power-washing of the old, lead-based paint on the exterior of the house prior to repainting. The fact that she used bare hands and then wiped them on her jeans before going inside the house is not a catastrophe, but it does illustrate how particles of lead move from the garden to the inside of homes where they may become airborne and at risk of being ingested when disturbed by the vacuum cleaner or broom. Kicking her boots off in the foyer is yet another reminder that lead in dirt literally walks right in our front doors.

We know the pre-renovation paint inside and outside the Millers' house contained lead by the age of the house and the fact that when they bought it, it had not been renovated. Based on its age, we can figure that the varying colors and layers of old paint contained approximately thirty percent lead. The fact that they disturbed it room by room over the duration of the renovation means for certain that considerable amounts of lead in the form of dust and paint chips have been circulating throughout the house. The dust in their house is undoubtedly toxic.

Sandy's handyman role in the nursery project exposed her needlessly to more of the chipping lead-based paint and construction dust that resulted. The removal of the lead paint in the baby's room was risky the way they went about it. Proper protection should have been worn and Sandy should have been out of the house completely. Instead, she helped scrape and sand. At least if the room had been sealed, the renovation would not have added as much lead to the house dust as this one did. Likewise, Sandy's proximity to the refinishing project in the basement, a project that employed large quantities of lead-containing furniture stripper, was an unfortunate and avoidable choice.

But neither the copious amounts of furniture stripper nor the old lead-based paint stripped from the baby's nursery raises the cause for concern that Craig's stained glass project does. Over a period of several weeks, Craig released lead vapor into the air inside the house as he soldered the old stained glass window back together. Had the Miller's had a toddler in the house during this time, a serious medical emergency may well have ensued. The lead soldering and the vapor released into the air increased the risk for significant damage to the Millers' baby's brain.

Had Sandy known that her favorite ceramic mug was glazed with lead-based toxins, she surely would have tossed it. The fact that she drank from it daily, and had for several years, makes it a factor in the overall picture of her lead exposure.

The Millers' house has been superficially upgraded and it is easy to forget that the original lead pipes, for example, remain intact. At some time in the house's history, bits of the plumbing were replaced and lead solder was used on copper plumbing, only partially solving the problem. Now, newly installed brass faucets in the bathrooms are the modern day culprit for lead. The newer they are, the more lead is released. If Sandy is not running the water to clear what is left in the pipes, particularly overnight or when they have been away from the house for the day, then their plumbing is a serious problem. She is needlessly exposing herself and her unborn child to damage from lead that will last a lifetime.

Any special occasion brings with it special jobs to do and traditions to follow. The sterling silver flatware that Sandy inherited from her grandmother was not a problem in itself. However, the silver polish she used on it was toxic with lead. The special once-a-year china would be eaten off, washed and put away, posing a small risk, a one-time short duration exposure. Better not to use it of course. However, the cut glass crystal stemware, filled with acidic juice and sipped slowly, posed a greater lead consumption risk.

When Craig lit the fire, he used the door and window moldings from upstairs as kindling. Their lead-based painted coatings burned off quickly in a blaze of exotic color, but also spewed dangerous lead fumes into the room. The colored inks from the wrapping paper that assisted with the starting of the fire similarly sent lead vapor into the surrounding room air.

Present Versus Past Exposure

In pregnancy, the fetus gathers materials it needs to build bone structure from the mother's bones. Lead from the maternal skeleton is transferred across the placenta to the fetus.[16] Later, additional lead exposure may occur during breast-feeding.[17] A critical factor in how much lead reaches the unborn baby is the amount of lead that has accumulated in the mother's bones over her lifetime. How much lead did Sandy Miller have in her bones and brain tissue prior to pregnancy? How much lead did she begin her life with at birth as a result of what her mother passed to her?

Sandy's father, like Craig, was connected to the petroleum industry and worked in a service station in town. The amount of lead that traveled into the home with Sandy's father would have significantly increased the family's lead accumulation over time. In the era of Sandy's childhood, we can count on the fact that the gasoline was leaded. And even if their house was the newest on the block, the math tells us that its paint would most certainly have been lead based.

But there is an equally large concern besides her father's occupation and the lead in the paint to which she was surely exposed in hazardous quantities. A nearby lead smelter puts this town on the map as a high-risk hotspot and puts Sandy Miller's probable bone lead levels precariously high.

The many sources of lead supplying seemingly insignificant amounts combine to a potentially devastating effect—brain damage which surfaces when a child begins to learn to read or needs to focus on a task. Suddenly, what went without notice or concern becomes a child's frustration in school and struggle throughout life.

NOTES

CHAPTER 3

BRINGING LEAD HOME

Once lead enters the environment, it remains in a perpetual cycle. Released into the atmosphere, it can travel long distances. Lead that has billowed from blast furnace chimneys in China, for example, drifts east to the North American continent. With the help of rain and gravity, airborne lead particles find their way into soil, dust and surface water. Since lead binds strongly with the particles of soil, it can remain in the upper soil layer for years. Particles which enter bodies of water become stuck to sediment for decades. In the areas where air, soil and water contain lead, it accumulates in plants and animals, changing into other forms, but never breaking down or disappearing.

Since the 1970s, some major sources of lead have been actively eliminated or reduced. The use of lead in house paint was phased out in 1977. Leaded plumbing solder and lead solder used in food cans were phased out in the 1980s. Lead was banned for use in gasoline for on-road motor vehicles in 1996. It is easy to be misled into thinking that because of these high-profile initiatives, the risk posed by lead has been minimized. On the contrary, we must not be deluded into thinking that the dangers of lead have been eradicated. Even today, lead can be found virtually everywhere, often in the least likely locations. It is as prevalent as ever.

An estimated forty percent of American housing contains some lead paint from applications made decades ago. Leaded fuel emissions that were deposited over the years in the soil near highways and train tracks continue the process of contamination. In some communities, lead-polluted water is still delivered through old lead pipes within the public water service. And despite all the talk about unleaded fuels, lead continues to fall from the sky as planes traverse over our heads.

There is no mistaking that lead is abundant in the environment surrounding us. But how does lead actually get into our homes and our bodies? As we might expect, much of it enters our homes via the air we breathe and water that comes through our faucets. But much of it comes home with us in shopping bags or is hauled to us in delivery trucks. Lead finds its way into our homes in our food supply, water, personal care products and in the toys we give to our children. Lead can be found on dinnerware, silverware, brassware and older pewterware. It lurks in crystals and plastics, in artwork and craft materials. It is used in the production of stained glass, jewelry, printing ink, dyes, candlewicks and cosmetics. It is found in bullets, shot, fishing nets and sinkers, in yachts and diving suits, curtain weights and emblems, in pipe organs and player pianos, in caulking and sound proofing materials, in ships, and in planes. The ever-growing electronics industry makes use of massive amounts of lead. Few people have any idea that a computer screen may contain as much as four pounds of this unwelcome metal.

Not only does lead find its way into our homes through the tap, in the air, and in the things that we buy for ourselves, lead travels on the tools, clothes, shoes, hair, skin and under the fingernails of people who are exposed while away from home. The sources of lead on jobsites and in the workplace are many and varied, making lead carried into the home by certain types of workers a significant household lead source.

Lead is everywhere, a silent hazard in our everyday lives. A vital part of minimizing exposure is knowing where to begin looking.

Lead in Food

Lead can contaminate food at any stage of harvesting, production, cooking, storage or distribution. It may enter from soil, as deposition from the air, or from contact with containers or food processing equipment. It can contaminate food via wrapping and labels. Regulation is the responsibility of government agencies such as the US Food and Drug Administration in the United States or the Food and Drug Act in Canada. In the United States, for example, the acceptable exposure to lead for children under six years of age has been set by the US Food and Drug Administration as less than six micrograms per day from all food sources, an amount that could easily be contained in one piece of lead-contaminated candy.

Candy produced in some foreign countries is at high risk for containing lead. Candy ingredients such as chili pepper and tamarind may be the source that introduces lead into candy. Imported candy is sometimes packaged in glazed clay pots that contain lead that eventually leaches into the product. Improper drying, storing and grinding during candy production increase the risk for lead exposure as well. Wrappers of both imported and domestic candies have been found to contain lead that eventually seeps into the treat.

Some amounts of lead in candy are allowed by the US Food and Drug Administration. The maximum permissible level of lead in candy has been established as 0.5 parts per million and since 2006 a recommended level of 0.1 parts per million has been suggested. As mentioned, the US Food and Drug Administration also recommends that children under age six consume less than six micrograms of lead each day from all food sources. In some cases, consuming just one candy can put youngsters above the recommended threshold. For example, one brand of candy imported from Mexico has been identified as containing as much as 0.3 to 0.4 micrograms of lead per gram of product. Since the average weight for one candy is thirty grams, by consuming just one candy a child could ingest nearly twice the recommended level.

It is not possible to tell if a candy contains lead by looking at it or tasting it. It is also hard to say which sweets contain what amounts of lead as they vary not only from candy to candy but also from batch to batch. As laboratory testing is required to establish that imported confectioneries are safe, the State of California passed Bill 121 in 2006 to ensure that large enough samples of available products are checked. This legislative initiative is unique to California where stores commonly carry candy from neighboring Mexico on their shelves and much of the population has a penchant for Mexican flavors.

Chocolate is a common hiding place for lead. There is debate as to whether the source of lead is sloppy manufacturing practices, the leaded gasoline used in farm equipment, or lead from fertilizers. Whatever the source of contamination, compared to other foods, chocolate contains higher amounts of lead. A study provided to the US Food and Drug Administration by the chocolate industry in 2005[18] analyzed 137 samples of milk chocolate and 226 samples of dark chocolate. It reported that milk chocolate contained as much as 0.222 parts per million of lead. With some samples containing up to 0.275 parts per million of lead, dark chocolate fared even worse. A fact sheet published by the American Environmental Safety Institute on lead in chocolate reports blood-lead increase caused by lead-containing chocolate in an average child of six years of age. Shockingly, the document[19] claims that a brand of chocolate fudge pudding (containing 2.7 micrograms of lead) results in a thirty-three percent increase in blood lead level. A cocoa drink (containing 3.67 micrograms of lead) results in a forty-five percent boost. A popular chocolate Easter bunny (containing 4.93 micrograms of lead) causes a sixty-one percent rise. Given what is known about lead exposure's effect of lowering IQ, and given the number of children who eat chocolate frequently, this is critical information for parents.

Canned food has contained high levels of lead in the past as a result of the use of lead-containing solder to seal seams on cans. This practice has been gradually phased out on the North American continent since the 1980s in favor of sealing by welding, or for certain foods, using tin solder. In 1991, US food canners voluntarily quit using lead solder. A complete, mandatory ban on lead solder used in canned goods produced in America, as well as in imported cans, was imposed by the US Food and Drug Administration in 1995.

Lead is still used, unfortunately, in cans that are imported from some foreign countries. It has been estimated by the US Food and Drug Administration that up to ten percent of imported food may be packaged in lead-soldered cans.[20] Foods, especially acidic ones, can leach lead from the solder in the cans' seams. When purchasing imported canned goods, look for one-piece cans with no side seam or cans sealed with a narrow seam line. Cans with a folded seam, usually with clip-like dents along the side, should be avoided. A black smudged line on the inside of a can is a certain indicator that lead solder was used and the food should not be consumed.

Tin-coated lead foil capsules on wine bottles were banned by the US Food and Drug Administration in 1996 after a study by the Bureau of Alcohol, Tobacco, and Firearms revealed that three to four percent of wines could become contaminated with lead residue from these capsules. Lead foils were used to prevent insect infestation and as an oxygen barrier. Often, wine became contaminated when it seeped between the cork and the foil wrap. Also, the corroded foil seal deposited lead contaminated residue on the rim of the bottle. The United States winemakers stopped using lead foils even before the ban, but older bottles with the foils may still be available.

Home gardens are a special problem for food contamination from lead. The romantic notion of growing healthy produce in the backyard might be safer to remain just that—a notion. Although we usually do not think of backyard gardens as dangerous places, much of our garden soil contains unsafe levels of lead. If garden plots are located on old industrial or commercial land or near industrial sources and highways, gardens will be contaminated. Soil contamination can also originate from weathered exterior paint and from homes that were power-washed and repainted if the original layers of paint were from the lead paint era.

Vegetable uptake of lead varies depending on the kind of produce. Lead does not readily accumulate in the fruiting part of vegetables and fruit. Thus, produce such as corn, beans, squash, okra, tomatoes, cucumbers, peppers, apples and berries are relatively safe. Unless soil lead levels are extremely high, most of the lead that is contained in produce comes from dust deposits rather than from plants' uptake of lead from soil. Higher concentrations of lead are more likely to be found in leafy greens such as lettuce, spinach and herbs. Root crops, including carrots, beets and potatoes, may also contain lead that they obtain from the soil. Lettuce, spinach, carrots, endives, cress and beetroots have been shown to have the highest uptake levels of lead.

Waterfowl and game may ingest or be killed with lead shot from hunters' guns. Now lead-poisoned, an animal may become sick or be consumed by unsuspecting hunters, their families or other animals that are a part of the food chain. Waterfowl may become poisoned from ingesting lead fishing sinkers.

Spices and seasoning originating from countries with inadequate regulations and control may be a risk. Contamination of herbs and spices can occur during growth in lead-contaminated soils, from lead containing pesticides, or during processing procedures such as drying using motors that run on leaded gasoline. The August 2005 issue of *Pediatrics* reported two incidents of childhood lead poisoning in families that used lead contaminated spices purchased in the Republic of Georgia and India. Also chili powder from Mexico has been reported to contain lead. For example, it has been found in lollipops coated with chili, as well as in a snack of a powdery mixture of salt, lemon flavor and chili seasoning.

Imported raisins may contain lead levels exceeding the US Food and Drug Administration's standard of 0.1 parts per million for lead in food. Some consignments of raisins available on the American and Canadian markets have tested to contain lead levels in excess of 0.25 parts per million.

Lead in Household Objects

The list of lead-containing products on store shelves is endless. Many, despite their lead content, are in compliance with existing regulations. Other items such as toys and furniture intended for children are in blatant violation of regulations and pose an extreme hazard to children. With much of North American production taking place in countries where there is cheaper labor, North American consumers are indirectly being subjected to the negative impact and risk posed by lower regulatory standards and insufficient monitoring.

Glazed ceramics, pottery and dishes are potential sources of dangerously high lead levels. Lead has been used in glazes for ceramic dishware since ancient times. Today, it is commonly used for the bright colors on ceramic dishes and to achieve a smooth, transparent glaze. However, if pottery with lead-containing glaze is not fired to a high enough temperature for a long enough time, lead will subsequently be released from the glaze into the food. The amount of lead that leaches depends on how the dish is used and what kind of food is put into it. Acidic foods and beverages such as tomato sauce, salad dressing, vinegar, fruit juice, coffee, wine and cola drinks should never be stored in or eaten out of dishes that contain lead. To illustrate the magnitude of the danger, a person drinking juice from lead-glazed pottery could be exposed to 135 micrograms daily.

If in doubt whether a dish contains lead, do not use it for food. The longer food stays in contact with a lead-containing dish, the more lead will leach into the food. Heating food also requires caution as higher temperature can speed up the leaching process. Repeated washing, cracks or scratches can cause leaded glazes to deteriorate.

Dishes and pottery made commercially in the United States, Canada and Western Europe are *generally* safe to use as they are made with lead free glazes, but consumers still need to ask and be cautious. Today many manufacturers of tableware maintain toll-free telephone lines where concerned consumers can have their questions about their product answered. Antiques and collectibles, dishes and pottery made in foreign countries, and pieces made by amateurs for gifts or craft fairs are far more likely to contain lead. Articles imported or brought from developing countries are unlikely to meet North American standards.

Crystal glassware and decanters can release lead into beverages. Ordinarily glassware does not contain lead; however, it is added to molten quartz to produce crystal that has greater strength and brilliance. The higher the lead content, the higher the quality of the crystal. Quality crystal may contain as much as thirty-two percent lead. In addition to the glass itself, the pigments used for decorating the lip rim area of glassware may contain lead-based pigment and pose an added risk of exposure.

Crystal glasses and decanters should never have beverages stored or served in them. Drinking from lead crystal glasses and bottles on a daily basis should be avoided and they should never be used for infants or children.

Crystals are also used in jewelry and as decorations on clothing. Some crystals, for example, contain lead added to create light refraction in the crystal. Lead also adds to the weight, thus giving the crystal a more substantial feel.

Pewter dishes or cups may contain lead depending on what combination of metals was used. Pewter is an alloy; it contains more than one metal. The kinds of metal used in pewter have changed over the years, as did the amounts of lead it contained. Today, lead is not used in the production of pewter, with tin and other metals used in its place. Modern pewter vessels do not contain lead and therefore can safely be used. A coloration of pewter will help determine if an item contains lead. If it is dark grey and tarnishes easily, one should assume it contains lead.

Espresso machines, coffee makers and imported kettles or urns may leach lead into water and beverages. The leaching is amplified by the use of hot water. For example, two models of espresso machine were recalled due to leaching excessive amounts of lead into coffee. Both models had built-in brass components that contained high amounts of lead in the alloy, and when the hot water came in contact with the brass, lead leached into the beverage. In June 2005, about 100,000 coffee makers were recalled because they could possibly leach lead into coffee.

Inexpensive or toy jewelry and accessories such as necklaces, pendants, bracelets, hair accessories, rings and key chains have become common recall items due to containing dangerous levels of lead. These items pose extreme hazard as they are often touched, put in the mouth, sucked on and swallowed. In March of 2006, a four-year-old boy died in Minneapolis as a result of swallowing a lead-containing charm. According to an advisory by Health Canada, lead is found in both imported and domestic-made jewelry.

Lead-containing items are of all shapes and sizes. Some of them may be metal plated while others are coated with enamel. Lead can be used in imitation pearls and vinyl cords. According to a survey conducted by the US Consumer Product Safety Commission,[21] metal parts in some products contained more than 500,000 parts per million of lead and some were as high as 950,000 parts per million. That equals fifty and ninety-five percent lead! An independent lab revealed lead levels of 20,000 parts per million in some vinyl cords on costume jewelry and 165,000 parts per million on a coating on a bracelet.[22]

In 2007, recalled items that were intended for use by children reached an all-time high. One million six hundred thousand Cub Scout totem badges, 695,200 rings, 4,182,300 bracelets, 374,250 necklaces, 311,000 children's sunglasses, 1,937,460 other jewelry, including various sets and combinations of rings, earrings, necklaces, bracelets and 561,000 key chains were recalled.[23] These soaring numbers potentially equal a devastating amount of lead exposure. What needs to be kept in mind is that recalling flawed items is one thing; keeping children away from lead's damage is another. Because an item has been recalled does not provide assurance that the lead has been removed or the item made safe. Due to variation in lead regulations across the world, what is deemed unsafe in one country can be legally shipped to other countries for resale.

Children's clothing that utilizes snap closures, buttons, zipper pulls, t-shirt transfers, and items made from heavy vinyl such as raincoats and boots may contain lead. Due to lead-containing paint, children's sunglasses often make it to the recall list as well (Go to http://www.cdc.gov/nceh/lead/Recalls/allhazards.htm for recall lists).

Colored ink on food wrappers, grocery store vegetable bags and on imported plastic bread bags may contain lead pigments that leach into food upon coming into contact.

Newspapers, magazines and books, before 1985, are often printed with lead-based inks. These materials should never be used as play objects or food wrapping.

Brass items such as musical instruments, bells, faucets, fittings and keys may contain lead. Brass is an alloy made from a combination of copper and zinc; since zinc and lead are mined together, zinc contains lead.

Keys may contain lead from two sources: as a natural contaminant of zinc and from lead added to brass to make the metal more durable. Even if keys are covered with a nickel coating, they are still not safe. The coating wears away and we are left touching lead-containing brass. Keys need to be kept away from children and never given as a toy. Pregnant women especially need to avoid holding keys for prolonged periods of time. Hands should be thoroughly washed after handling keys.

Piano keys may be inserted with lead weights to achieve more volume. By depressing a key in the low bass register and checking the area under the wood part of the adjacent key, these weights can be detected. Frequent use may generate dust, which could end up on the fingers and in the mouths and lungs of children.

Bathtubs, especially older ones, may contain as much as eighty-eight percent lead in their glaze. Although lead uptake through the skin is minimal, lead from the bathtub can be absorbed if the skin is broken as in the case of cuts and scratches, or it can be ingested by children who drink bath water. The amount of leached lead increases when the enamel becomes cracked, chipped or worn.

Soundproofing materials may include lead. Since it is an excellent acoustical barrier, lead particles and sheets are commonly used. Sound insulation can be found in places such as between floor levels and rooms, in home theaters and music studios.

Vinyl products contain lead that is used in Polyvinyl Chloride, PVC. Lead softens plastic and increases its flexibility, as well as stabilizes molecules from heat. When exposed to elements such as sunlight, air and detergents, the bond between plastic and lead is severed and lead-containing dust is formed. This dust can be passed from hands to mouth or inhaled.

Lunchboxes used by children were recently in the news because of their discovered lead content. Food that has been stored in these particular lead containing lunchboxes may absorb the lead. Another possible source of exposure is when children touch lunchboxes with their hands and then handle their food. In a study conducted by government scientists, one in five lunchboxes (twenty percent) contained amounts of lead that are considered unsafe for children; more than 600 parts per million (0.06 percent). Some of them contained lead levels more than ten times that considered hazardous. The highest level measured was 9600 parts per million, more than sixteen times the acceptable standard.[24]

An ironic incident involving lunchboxes and lead took place when the California Department of Public Health distributed more than 50,000 lunchboxes with slogans such as "Eat Fruits & Vegetables and be Active." As was discovered later, the promotional lunchboxes included excessive amounts of lead. Accordingly, the organization asked the consumers not to use them and urged Californians to keep the lunchboxes away from infants and young children.

Baby bibs made of vinyl have been reported to contain lead, of particular concern when they are worn and cracked. However, as small children are prone to chew and suck, even new bibs pose a potential threat of lead exposure. Like toys, these lead-containing bibs have been sold by major retailers. Some contained as much as 9700 parts per million; an amount sixteen times greater than the legal limit of lead in paint.[25]

Vinyl mini-blinds imported from China, Taiwan, Mexico and Indonesia may pose a lead poisoning hazard. According to the US National Safety Council, twenty-five million mini-blinds available on the North American market are imported annually from these countries.[26] These non-glossy blinds have lead added to stabilize the plastic. Due to exposure to sunlight and heat over time, the plastic deteriorates and forms lead dust on the surface of the blind. Washing the blinds does not prevent the hazard of lead exposure. Blinds are available that specify that they are lead free.

Christmas light strands are almost always made using lead. This includes the new energy saving LED (light-emitting diode) lights. Manufacturers use lead in the PVC coating that insulates Christmas light wiring. Lead is used legally as a fire retardant and to prolong the longevity of the lights. Children should be kept away from Christmas light wiring and adults should wash hands and clothing after handling light strands.

Artificial Christmas trees can pose a risk of lead poisoning according to the University of North Carolina-Ashville Environmental Studies Department.[27] In a sample of artificial trees tested, one-fourth contained high levels of lead. Some practical advice offered by the researchers to those who want to avoid lead poisoning from their Christmas tree included keeping children away from the tree, washing hands after touching it, and avoiding vacuuming under the tree unless the vacuum is specifically designed with a High Efficiency Particulate Air (HEPA) filter.

Garden hoses can accumulate lead that either leaches from the vinyl contained in the hose or from the brass nozzle. Lead is of particular concern on hot days because as the hose becomes hot from the sunshine it leaches more lead. When buying a hose, check that the label states specifically that it is safe to drink from. All hoses should be flushed before use.

Curtain weights need to be kept out of children's reach. If swallowed, lead weights can cause poisoning or death.

Imported crayons and sidewalk chalk are often tainted with lead. Imported products should be avoided. North American–made alternatives that are specifically non-toxic are available.

Billiard chalk has been found to contain precariously high lead levels; up to 7000 parts per million.[28] Lead is used as a coloring agent in this product. Pool cue chalk has been reported as a cause of lead poisoning in children. Children can be exposed to it by either chewing on the chalk or from the dust it deposits in the house.

Electronics contain large amounts of lead. It can be found in solder, various plated surfaces, in circuit boards and plastic elements. Only between five to ten percent of personal use products such as cellular phones, TVs, cameras or radios are made using lead-free components.[29] Lead content in these products does not pose immediate danger, especially when they are in good repair. But when no longer in use, this electronic waste is a huge problem. So far, unlike the European Union, the United States has not adopted consistent regulations pertaining to e-waste. Most of it ends up on far-away continents such as Africa or Asia.

Candlewicks may utilize lead as a stiffener. Lead becomes absorbed by inhalation while burning candles with lead core wicks. Lead-containing wicks are usually used in candles that are intended for longer burning, such as ceremonial or scented candles. In 1974, the candle industry agreed with the US Consumer Product Safety Commission to voluntarily stop making candles with lead-containing wicks; however, wicks in candles imported from other countries and some candles made in Canada and in the United States may still contain lead. According to Health Canada, an estimated ten percent of candles available on the Canadian market contain lead core wicks. A candle can be tested for lead by separating the wick's fiber strands to see if there is a metallic core inside. When the metallic core is rubbed on a piece of white paper, a grey mark indicates lead.

Furniture imported from other countries often contains excessive amounts of lead. Even cribs and other furniture intended for use by children are not always lead free. On the contrary, it is usually items used by children that are the object of massive recalls (Go to http://www.cdc.gov/nceh/lead/Recalls/allhazards.htm for recall lists). Antiques and pieces handed down from generation to generation should also raise concern.

Tobacco smoke contains lead, mainly from the arsenate pesticides that are found in cigarettes. Obviously, cigarette smoking or inhaling of second-hand smoke increases exposure to lead.

Pets pick up and carry lead dust on their paws and coats. Animal fur can collect and redistribute substantial amounts of lead.

Lead in Toys

Antique toys should immediately raise a concern. Their age tells us that they were made when lead was not recognized as a hazard or regulated. Today, even though the dangers that lead poses to children are well known and documented, lead-laced toys still find their way to store shelves. Toy recalls have increased steadily in the past three decades and recently have become daily headlines in the news.

Contrary to a previous assumption that only cheaply made toys sold at discount stores contain lead, the issue affects nearly all popular toy chains. Trusted toy manufacturers have recently had to recall millions of toys. In June of 2007, 1.5 million wooden railways were recalled because of lead paint. Three months later, more than half a million Chinese-made products met the same fate with 544,000 products recalled due to their lead content. While some recalled products such as cups, key chains, bookmarks and journals contained lead in their surface paint, others had lead imbedded in the material structure itself (Go to http://www.cdc.gov/nceh/lead/Recalls/allhazards.htm for recall lists).

The US Consumer Products Safety Commission urges buyers to become educated about safety when buying toys and to check warning labels carefully. Toy labels, however, rarely if ever disclose that they contain lead. Furthermore, disposing of toys containing lead is a challenge.

Lead in Personal Care Products and Cosmetics

More and more studies report that lead and other common cosmetic ingredients play a role in a host of long-term health problems that go beyond neurological damage to include cancer and infertility. The lack of knowledge about the effects that combining these different ingredients may have is a growing concern. David Baltz, a scientist with Commonwealth, a California-based non-profit health and environmental research institute, says that the general regulatory structure of chemicals is grossly inadequate worldwide. According to Baltz, most chemical ingredients receive their approval for use in commerce with very little or no testing for safety; they are presumed safe until proven otherwise. The Environmental Working Group, a Washington-based organization which co-ordinates activist campaigns on consumer products, reveals that of the 10,500 chemical ingredients used in personal-care products, a mere eleven percent have been tested by a government body for safety. The organization claims the remaining eighty-nine percent of untested ingredients are used in more than ninety-nine percent of all products on the market.

Lipstick produced by top brand companies has been reported to contain lead. While it is possible to make lipstick without lead, the tests conducted by the Campaign for Safe Cosmetics[30] suggest that lipstick manufactured in the United States and used daily by millions of women may contain lead. Of thirty-three top-brand North American lipsticks tested, sixty-one percent contained detectable levels of lead. One-third of the lipsticks exceeded 0.1 parts per million, the Food and Drug Administration's limit for lead in candy, a seemingly small amount, but one that compounds quickly as it is used and ingested on a regular or daily basis. According to some estimates, the average woman will swallow *pounds* of lipstick in a lifetime. Lead finds its way into lipstick either as a pigment or it may be a by-product from ingredients that come from raw materials such as zinc oxide and titanium dioxide, mineral wax or paraffin and petroleum-based ingredients. The US Food and Drug Administration has yet to establish a lead limit for cosmetics.

Eye cosmetics made using powders, gels or water-based fluids imported from the Indian subcontinent and Middle East are potential sources of lead. Significant amounts of lead can be absorbed from cosmetic eye products (see appendix 4).

Hair dye ingredients used in products such as progressive hair dyes which gradually color the hair or disguise grey hair often contain lead acetate. Despite the fact that the US Food and Drug Administration considers these products safe for use, it requires that the manufacturer place the following warning on the product:

> Caution: Contains lead acetate. For external use only. Keep this product out of children's reach. Do not use on cut or abraded scalp. If skin irritation develops, discontinue use. Do not use to color mustaches, eyelashes, eyebrows, or hair on parts of the body other than the scalp. Do not get in eyes. Follow instructions carefully and wash hands thoroughly after use.

Henna hair dying products vary. While natural henna is made from the henna plant and does not contain any chemical additives, other products labeled henna may contain lead acetate. These dyes deposit lead sulfide and lead oxide on the hair.

Powder, baby talcum and baby creams may contain lead that usually comes from the active ingredient, zinc oxide. Zinc oxide, widely used to treat skin irritations, is often contaminated with lead. Even though lead does not easily penetrate healthy skin, once applied to sensitive areas of irritated or broken skin, such as babies' diaper rash, it is readily absorbed.

Calcium supplements that come from natural sources may contain lead. Considerable quantities of lead have been found in some over-the-counter calcium supplement preparations, including bone meal, dolomite and some natural and refined calcium carbonate formulations. Calcium that is derived from such natural sources as dolomitic limestone and oyster shells has become commonly contaminated by lead. Ironically, products that are advertised as "all natural" frequently contain the highest levels of lead. Some supplements that are specifically lead free are available.

Diarrhea relief medications have been found to contain high lead levels. For over fifty years, popular brands of anti-diarrheals have been used freely by both pregnant women and children. Those formulas which are based on the ingredient, attapulgite clay, contain high levels of lead. Recently, one manufacturer was ordered by a court decision to lower lead levels in their anti diarrheal product. That same company announced that they would remove lead completely and replace it with bismuth subsalicylate, an ingredient used in stomach remedies.

Folk remedies containing lead have been used in many cultures since ancient times. Today, these remedies continue to be used in developing nations. Lead may be contained in folk remedies used by Hispanic, East Indian, Indian, Middle Eastern and West Asian populations. Some remedies contain lead that is added to the remedy purposefully in the belief that it enhances healing properties. In others, lead finds its way into the remedy as a contaminant during production. These remedies are brought by immigrants to their new countries where a new demand is created. They are sold in ethnic stores and by folk healers. It is speculated that each year these remedies cause thousands of cases of lead poisoning that result in either illness or death. According to the US Centers for Disease Control and Prevention, traditional remedies may account for up to thirty percent of cases of lead poisoning in children in the United States. Many cases, especially the ones involving lower level exposure, go unreported. Lead poisoning has been linked to herb medicine, baby tonics, teething powder, bone meals, aphrodisiacs and various ointments, some of them containing as much as ninety percent of lead (see appendix 4).

Lead in Drinking Water

The amount of lead contained in the water depends on the materials used in the pipes and the amount of wear in them, how long the water stays in the pipes, its temperature, acidity, as well as the types and amounts of minerals present in the water.

Some drinking water systems may present a lead exposure hazard. In the early part of the twentieth century, the main sources of water contamination were water pipes in homes and water storage tanks. Today, lead pipes remain in use underground as service lines in many older communities. In the 1980s, lead solder that was used in the process of joining copper pipes was found to be a source of lead in drinking water. In later years, water that came from soldered water coolers was identified as containing high lead levels.

Lead leaches into drinking water not only from lead pipes and the solder on copper pipes but also in some cases from PVC pipes. Brass plumbing materials, such as faucets and some water meters and well-pump components may contain as much as eight percent lead.

In recent years, a combination of bismuth and selenium has been developed as a substitute for traditional plumbing components. Although trace amounts of lead are still present in this combination, they are considered "lead-free" in the plumbing industry.

Today, the US Environmental Protection Agency estimates that up to twenty percent of a child's total lead exposure is attributed to lead-contaminated water. Formula-fed infants are at significant risk. In order to ensure that our children are not drinking lead-contaminated water, lead levels should be checked not only in homes but also at schools and daycares where children spend prolonged periods of time. Pregnant women especially should take care to avoid water that contains lead, since lead crosses the placenta to the unborn child.

Although there is no "safe" level of lead in water, the US Environmental Protection Agency has established an "action level" for lead in drinking water at fifteen parts per billion.

Compared to cold water, hot water increases the amount of leached lead. Accordingly, cooking with hot water obtained from the tap should be rigorously avoided. Lead reaches its highest levels in water left in pipes that has sat for many hours or overnight. However, even two hours or less is enough for water to accumulate concerning amounts of lead. In order to avoid ingesting contaminated water, "flushing" for at least thirty seconds to a minute prior to using it for cooking or drinking is critical.

In 2001, CBC's investigative consumer program, *Marketplace,* tested water from fifty homes across Canada. Water samples came from Saint John, Toronto, Hamilton, Winnipeg and Vancouver. Half of the tested water came from houses built before 1970 and half were built after. Only fifteen of the tested homes had lead levels at the national guideline of ten micrograms per litre. Water in the remaining thirty-five houses exceeded the national standard. One house had levels 250 times the allowable limit. The highest contamination levels were detected in water that came from houses built before 1970. In general, older houses are believed to pose the highest risk for lead exposure from plumbing, but as lead may leach from new solder for several years, brand new construction also presents lead dangers.

Occupational Lead Exposure

Occupational exposure is a significant source of lead. Individuals working in construction, home renovation, steel and bridgework, and other industries that use lead bring home lead dust on their clothes, shoes, skin and hair. The interior of the vehicles they drive may become contaminated with lead. As a result, jobs which involve lead exposure may impact not only the individual directly engaged in the profession, but also their spouses and children. For example, a study conducted amongst workers in the lead battery industry discovered that lead dust transported home on their clothes, shoes and hair contributed significantly to the lead loads of their children. Twelve out of sixteen children of the battery workers had elevated blood levels of lead.[31]

Occupations Associated with Lead Exposure

Aircraft repair
Auto body painting
Automotive body repair
Automotive radiator repair
Battery manufacturing
Battery breaking
Battery recycling
Brass manufacturing
Bridge construction
Building maintenance
Bridge repair
Cable repair
Cable stripping
Ceramic glaze mixing
Ceramics making
Chemical industry
Closed-wheel auto racing
Commercial painting
Commercial remodeling
Commercial renovation
Construction demolition
Construction work
Copper production
Demolition of ships
Driving on major highways
Electrical
Electronics welding
Elevated highway construction
Firearms instruction
Firing range
Fishing
Foundry work
Furniture refinishing
Gas station work
Gasoline additives production
Glass manufacturing
Glaze mixing
Home remodeling
Home renovation
Industrial painting
Ironwork
Jewelry-making
Lead abatement work

Lead mining
Lead processing
Lead smelting
Locksmithing
Machine manufacturing
Machining and grinding
Mechanics
Metalwork
Mining
Paint manufacturing
Painting
Pigment manufacturing
Pipe fitting
Police work involving firearms
Plastic industry
Plumbing
Pottery making
Printing
Radiator manufacturing
Radiator repair
Recycling operations
Refinery work
Roofing
Rubber industry
Scrap metal handling
Sandblasting
Sanding of oil paint
Scrap metal industry
Shellac manufacturing
Shipbuilding
Ship-fitting
Ship work
Smelting
Soldering of lead products
Solid waste production
Stained glass making
Steel bridge maintenance
Steel welding and cutting
Thermal pain stripping
Tunnel construction
Welding
X-ray shielding

Art supplies may contain lead. Although lead has been removed from most art materials, it can still be contained in "flake white" colors, in chromate colors and in many pigments. Individuals purchasing materials need to be especially vigilant and thorough in their research to find safe alternative paint product. The common practice of stopping for lunch or meal break with paint still on the artist's hands and clothing greatly increases the risk of ingestion, a factor frequently cited in considering the many toxin-related afflictions that painters and artists have suffered for ages.

Firing ranges are a source of dangerous exposures to lead. Lead dust is produced from abrasion of bullets as they pass through the gun barrel and from fragments created when bullets strike the backstop. Lead residues remain on shell casings that are often collected for reloading. Since lead dust clings to clothing, shoes and accessories worn or used at the range, the families of persons who work at or use firing ranges are also subject to "take-home" exposure to lead. The closure of a day-care center in Clearwater, Florida illustrates how lead residue can become transient and cause harm. When it was discovered that lead from a nearby indoor shooting range was drifting into the center's playground area, the day-care center was forced to close.[32]

Fishing may provide instances of lead exposure. Most fishing weights and sinkers are made from lead. Non-lead alternatives are becoming increasingly available.

Lead figurines are statues cast primarily of lead and accordingly have been identified as a potential source. They include military and fantasy figurines that are sold in huge numbers as collectibles or game pieces. They can be bought at hobby shops, comic book stores, craft fairs and toy stores.

Car racing exposes racing crews, other staff and spectators to lead from the fuel. In a letter from the president of the group Clean Air Watch, to the chairman and CEO of NASCAR, he wrote,

> By permitting the continued use of lead, your organization may be putting millions of spectators and nearby residents at unnecessary risk of suffering serious health effects.[33]

The US Environmental Protection Agency has noted that lead particles from auto exhaust can remain drifting in the air for more than a week, ending up many miles from its original source.

NASCAR reports that they have been researching alternative racing fuels that, until now, caused damage to racing engines. A new lead free formulation has recently been under development. Although NASCAR has recently announced that the new unleaded fuel will be used in major races, the racing community is not entirely pleased. In Canada, members of parliament have received an on-line petition against the move to ban leaded fuels on the racetrack. One protester commented,

> This is like a $200-million hit for the racing industry in Canada and I'm hoping we're getting the government's attention. I believe once they see the financial impact and the general interest of the public, they will have to take another look at this.[34]

Unfortunately, vehicles designed for speed have not been alone in maintaining a demand for leaded fuels. Some off-road vehicles such as those that perform for large enclosed audiences, farm equipment and marine engines have continued to use leaded fuel.

Hobbies Associated with Lead Exposure

Ammunition making
Automotive
Antique furniture restoration
Antique toys, soldiers, figurines
collecting and restoration
Battery work
Billiards (lead in cue chalk)
Boat building
Boat repair
Brass work
Bronze casting
Casting bullets
Casting lead pewter
Casting lead shot
Car racing
Ceramics making
Clothing accessory making
Coin collecting
Collecting lead toys and figurines
Copper enameling
Diving (lead in diving weights and
other gear)
Explosives work
Fishing
Fishing tackle making
Furniture stripping and refinishing
Glass art
Glass blowing using leaded glass
Glazing

Jewelry making
Lead lighting
Lead soldering
Mechanics
Metal miniature making
Mineral specimen art mosaics
Model car making
Old toy restoration
Painting using lead-based artists' paints
Pastel art
Pewter work
Pottery
Printmaking
Radiator maintenance
Radiator repair
Reloading shells
Remodeling
Renovation
Soldering of electronics
Stained glass artistry
Target shooting at firing ranges
'War games' model making
Welding

Lead in Paint

Paint remains a leading contaminator and lead exposure source. Lead was added to oil and some latex paint for pigmentation and as a drying agent. Despite the fact that in 1978 the limit of lead in interior paint was lowered to 0.06 percent, lead paint still abounds in older houses. Since young children often put their fingers and objects in their mouths, they can be easily poisoned by ingesting lead that comes either from paint chips and particles or house dust. The ban that prohibits the use of leaded paint pertains to house paint, toys and articles intended for use by children. Other things included in the ban include furniture such as beds, chests, bookcases and tables. It does not apply to paint on appliances such as ranges, refrigerators and washers. It also excludes fixtures such as built-in-cabinets, windows, doors and household products such as blinds and shades.

Industrial paint continues to pose a serious, ongoing problem. Lead-containing paint used for industrial and agricultural structures, building and equipment maintenance and billboards and road signs is allowed. It is permitted in lawn and garden equipment and on radio-controlled model airplanes. Unlike the aforementioned products that require specific warning on their labels, products such as mirrors with leaded backing paint and metal furniture that is not intended for use by children require no labeling.

Lead-containing paint is favored for its ability to expand and contract with a metal surface without cracking, as well as its resistance to corrosion. If eaten or digested, chips and dust derived leaded paint pose a serious health risk. Also the stripping and sanding of old paint produce lead particles that can be inhaled and swallowed. The practice of power-washing homes before repainting has greatly increased soil and yard contamination where chips of lead-containing paint are loosened and scattered.

Lead in Soil

Bare soil invariably contains lead that was either deposited in the past by vehicle emissions or old paint, or it originates from current releases such as pesticides and hobbies that use lead. This is especially true in the case of vacant lots where old buildings once stood or neighborhoods where extensive renovations took place. Since average intestinal absorption of lead in children is five times greater that in adults, the most critical exposure to lead contained in soil occurs when the contaminated soil or dust end up in children's mouths.

Lead in Dust

Dust formed from lead-containing paint is easily absorbed and is the most common source of lead exposure. Lead in dust may originate from deteriorating interior paint, soil and from fallout of airborne lead particles from industrial use. Lead-containing dust accumulates on furniture, floors and carpets. It finds its way into children's toys, bedding and clothing. Its particles enter the human body either by being inhaled as lead-polluted air or ingested as lead particles from various household objects. The amount of lead contained in the air correlates directly with the blood-lead levels; it is more predictive of elevated blood-lead levels than the amount of lead contained in the house paint.[35]

Renovation, Remodeling and Lead

Renovation and remodelling activities are the chief producers of lead-contaminated dust. Consequently, they are a significant contributor to both the number of identified cases of lead poisoning and unrealized exposure. Before any renovation or remodelling activities, it is important to be aware of the potential presence of lead in paint applied before it was banned.

Lead also hides in construction materials such as sealants, caulk and lead putty. Sealants are usually applied around sinks, bathtubs, as well as around windows and doors, while cracks and gaps in wood and walls are patched with lead-containing caulking. Lead putty can be used to fill undesired cracks and holes. Unfortunately, with time this product tends to crumble and flake, thus creating a lead exposure hazard.

Lead on Playground Equipment

Playground equipment can be a source of lead exposure, especially where there is chipping and peeling lead paint. Lead can be ingested as paint particles, chips and dust transfer from children's hands to their mouths. In a recent study conducted by the US Consumer Product Safety Commission, twenty-six playgrounds located in thirteen different cities were evaluated. Sixteen playgrounds had lead levels high enough to be recognized as a federal priority for lead hazard control action.

It is no longer possible to rest on our laurels assuming that in this modern world the potential for lead exposure has been minimized through the many steps that the government and the manufacturers have already taken. After all, the facts of lead's harm have been known for long enough. The work still to be done is substantial. Compound ongoing sources of lead with the lead of yesterday still with us, lead remains pervasive.

It is more important than ever that we appreciate the gravity of the issue, not only its astounding prevalence but also our own susceptibility to lead's harm. Fortunately, once we fully appreciate these realities, the steps that follow, are encouraging.

NOTES

CHAPTER 4

LEAD AND TODDLERS: THE BLOOD-BRAIN BARRIER

Children are not small versions of adults. In comparison, children drink more fluids, eat more food, breathe more air relative to body weight, and have a larger skin surface in proportion to their body volume.[36] As a result, babies and toddlers are at a far greater risk for experiencing lead-induced health effects than older children and adults.

There are a number of specific examples of how differences come into play relative to lead exposure risk. To begin with, babies and toddlers have been documented to absorb lead via the gastrointestinal tract more efficiently (fifty percent relative absorption) than adults (fifteen percent relative absorption).[37] They do not typically consume the same foods as their parents in the first years of life, and consequently, the result is a greater prevalence of nutrient deficiency.[38] The diets of young children, for example, are not uncommonly deficient in zinc, a condition that exacerbates the toxic effects of lead. Dietary deficiencies of calcium and iron, common in children, have also been shown to increase the risk of lead poisoning.[39] Thus, there is broad consensus that nutrient deficiencies in children at high-risk stages of neurological development put these children at a substantially elevated risk for lead-related injury in comparison to their parents, caregivers and older siblings.

Young children have also been shown to have lower blood thresholds for the hematological (blood-related) and neurological (brain-related) effects induced by lead exposure, while the resultant brain injuries and central nervous system deficits tend to be much more severe.[40] Consideration of these differences begins to build an appreciation for a baby or toddler's susceptibility and vulnerability to lead. Recognizing these differences is the key to planning for and providing adequate protection.

Susceptibility to lead exposure changes with age. The likelihood of lead exposure has to do with the way in which individuals interact with their environment, varying greatly as children progress from newborn through sitting up, crawling and eventually walking. Crawling children will experience lead sources that walking children or adults may not come in contact with. Children who have pacifiers or suck their thumbs are overall more likely to be exposed to lead than children who put their hands in their mouths less. Children who play in the dirt or sand outdoors may become exposed to lead that adults protected by gloves will avoid.

A child's vulnerability will depend to a great extent on the developmental stage at the time of exposure. Just as there are critical periods of structural and functional development in the prenatal life of a child, postnatal growth and development of the central nervous system are also key.[41] Consideration of our own nervous systems as adults will illustrate the important contrast in vulnerability between that of a small child and someone beyond the threshold of development of those first two years of life. The difference is an extremely important point when trying to understand why lead does such a disproportionate amount of damage to the youngest brains.

For the sake of comparison, imagine that the adult brain is a coconut. A thick green husk and a hard inner shell provide a layer of protection for the white meat and milk contained inside. Like the coconut meat, the human brain is protected physically by the hard bone of a skull. This shield protects not only from a bump on the head but also from chemical toxins. This protective layer is something we call the blood-brain barrier, and with the exterior armor of the skull, the brain is the best-protected part in the adult body. By comparison to other vulnerable organs and systems in the body, the command center of the nervous system housed in the adult human skull is all but cut off from the outside world, enjoying protection that the liver, kidneys, gastrointestinal and respiratory systems do not.

The central nervous system has no such protection when it is in its formative stages, and to complicate the matter, this highly vulnerable unprotected developmental phase continues for a full two years after a child is born. The first six months after birth, even longer if the birth is premature, is a period of extreme vulnerability. The brain is literally still under construction. This is followed by a second phase that continues until around age two. This is a delicate period of fine-tuning when the synaptic connections between neurons are established. Around the child's second birthday, the system prunes itself, reducing the number of synaptic connections that have thus far been established, by half.

The fact that the brain undergoes critical phases of development well after birth prolongs the window of vulnerability. This is further impacted by the fact that a baby's head is not hard like a coconut, and by the fact that the blood-brain barrier, which the adult nervous system enjoys as a critical layer of protection, is not formed right away. We can best characterize the time from birth until twenty-four months as a dangerously critical time for exposure to even the lowest measurable levels of lead.

The egg given to partnered teens to care for over an assigned sequence of days in the well-known parenthood exercise offers a very appropriate metaphor for the vulnerability of a newborn. For if an adult's brain is strong like a coconut, then the infant's is fragile like an egg. Keeping the egg safe from harm is a very unforgiving endeavor. The difference between the egg exercise and real life is that even though the parents may succeed in not *dropping* their egg, allowing it to be exposed to a long list of lead sources may do irreparable damage to the part of the egg they cannot actually see.

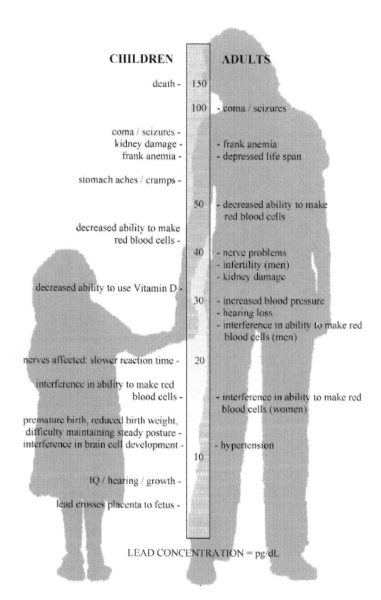

CHILDREN   ADULTS

death -	150
	100 - coma / seizures
coma / seizures - kidney damage - frank anemia -	- frank anemia - depressed life span
stomach aches / cramps -	
	50 - decreased ability to make red blood cells
decreased ability to make red blood cells -	
	40 - nerve problems - infertility (men) - kidney damage
decreased ability to use Vitamin D -	
	30 - increased blood pressure - hearing loss - interference in ability to make red blood cells (men)
nerves affected: slower reaction time -	20
interference in ability to make red blood cells -	- interference in ability to make red blood cells (women)
premature birth, reduced birth weight, difficulty maintaining steady posture - interference in brain cell development -	- hypertension
	10
IQ / hearing / growth -	
lead crosses placenta to fetus -	

LEAD CONCENTRATION = pg/dL

Children and adults do not experience the effects of lead equally.
Children are impacted earlier and more severely than adults.
Adapted from ATSDR, Toxicological Profile for Lead, 1989

Bill Richardson mentally went through the list of things he was supposed to have picked up from the store as he swung his car into the driveway. Satisfied that he had everything—the cake, the balloon bouquet and red wrapping paper—he turned off the ignition. He then turned his attention to a new list of chores that was quickly mounting in his head as he looked at the flowerbeds, the lawn and edging. And then to almost two-year-old Molly.

As per usual, she was standing at the living room window, window ajar, calling hello. Ever since she had discovered she could pull herself up to standing, this was her favorite place to do it. She would watch out the window, sometimes forever it seemed, mesmerized by the mere prospect of a bike going by, a cat crossing the yard, or best of all, the arrival of her father's car. If she wasn't at the window waiting, there was usually a bit of drool left where she had been minutes earlier, teething quietly at her perch. As she had grown a bit and learned to stabilize her balance, the low wide sill became a favorite place for her and teddy to sip pretend tea together, or share a cookie.

Time had passed quickly, Bill realized as he waved to her from the driveway. Tomorrow's family birthday celebration would mark the milestone of two whole years. He would be forty this year himself—his second marriage. With his arms full of the cake box and his head being pummeled by eight tethered red balloons, he couldn't decide if this milestone was making him feel young or old. At least, he thought as he looked around the tiled entry foyer, there were no renovations required in this house. The previous owners had done that for them, and essentially, apart from the age of the foundation and framing, the house felt new.

Before Bill finished his thought, the cat wandered between his legs, followed immediately, also on all fours, by Molly. Looking up at him was a round pink face and red curls that he recognized, but a set of cat whiskers that he didn't. As she proclaimed herself a cat and meowed off after the family pet, Bill's wife, Jennifer, arrived from the dining room to explain that there had been face painters at the park that afternoon, and Molly had insisted.

The next day was Saturday and first thing, Bill was up and out in the yard in anticipation of the upcoming afternoon events. Once the lawn was cut and the mower put away, Molly joined him in the yard to "help."

The day before, a few areas in the walkway had been spot-sprayed for weeds, and now he plucked at the withered remains before sweeping up. From the corner of his eye, he noticed Molly lingering where he had the hose watering a flowerbed. Sure enough, before he could get to her, she had the hose to her mouth and water splattering in every direction. He whisked it out of her hand before she was soaked, and relocated her to the swing set on the other side of the yard. He helped her wipe her wet hands off on a partially wet t-shirt. It had a picture of Elmo on it that said "Molly is two." Jennifer laughed at the predictability of it all as she finished tying the balloons to the aluminum railing on the back deck and then disappeared inside the house to get food ready for the party.

Molly had no interest in swinging and was instantly back at Bill's side with her hands in the soil that he was attempting to run a rake over. When he told her to stop she ignored him, and when he physically removed her she kicked and screamed. Typically a delightful and compliant little girl, Molly seemed less and less so lately. Today he and Jennifer waved it off as due to all the excitement of the birthday party. Bill fetched a plastic children's rake from the shed and they took short shifts in the garden until that was no longer interesting and Molly sauntered off to bother the cat. The truth of the matter was, practically overnight, Molly had become hyperactive and difficult to manage.

The party began at the tail end of Molly's afternoon nap. The in-laws arrived in fancy sundress and old man shorts. Jennifer's sister and brother-in-law pulled in with the only three other kids invited. Jonathan, twelve, would be hooked to his iPod, and five-year-old twins, Amy and Sarah, would be stereo nannies for Molly if all went as planned.

The video camera was fully charged and on standby when Molly's two little candles were lit. Someone thought it would be cute for Molly to wear one of the big red bows off the present she was opening, but she tore it off her head unappreciatively and let them know the scotch tape pulled her hair. Nonetheless, the progress from last year was notable. She tore the paper off her gifts, but this year she played with several of the gifts, rather than the wrapping paper that was wholly the object of her fascination during year one's festivities. In honor of the special occasion, her grandparents presented her with an antique pewter cup that had been in the family for three generations. They insisted that it was hers to use and filled it with a scoop of juice from the punch bowl.

The red theme felt a bit like a celebration of Chinese New Year, but it was Molly's favorite color. There were brightly colored tablecloths, paper plates, cups and napkins. The celebration came to a crescendo about the time that the last of the presents was opened and the bottom of the punch bowl appeared.

The twins had spent the afternoon sitting happily on the walkway with a set of jacks that Jennifer had put in a goody-bag for them. Maybe it was the Smarties and jujubes that were in the bag that kept them content. Either way, they never bothered anyone, and Bill wondered what it would take to grow his cantankerous Molly into an approximation of these two sweet little girls. His wife and her sister had somewhat similar personalities and many shared traits. Perhaps the twins were as miserable at two as Molly, and she would outgrow this. Maybe the terrible twos would pass and life would be normal again.

Bill and Jennifer Richardson are caring parents providing the kind of stimulation and opportunity that good parenting books write about. The notion that lead poisoning is an affliction of the poor is an outdated assumption, but so is the idea that their house is safe because it is new or has been completely renovated to look and feel like new.

The windowsill that Molly first pulled herself up on as a baby, and now plays at daily, is a potential lead hazard. If it has been repainted, the danger lies in the fact that the daily repeated opening and closing creates lead-contaminated dust. It would be an important site in the house to check. Molly teethed at this spot as babies so typically do and has had toys and cookies on the sill collecting up leaded dust, which is at very least coming in contact with Molly's skin, and more likely actually being ingested. An accumulated amount of lead equal to three granules of table sugar would be enough to cause permanent neurological damage to a child Molly's size and age.

Pets with fluffy coats are always agents of transfer, bringing in trace amounts of lead in outdoor dust on their fur and paws to add to the collective household deposits. The fluffier the animal the more of a contributor. And the painted-on cat whiskers? Face paint, especially cheap imported kids' stuff, is notorious for containing lead.

Garden hoses frequently contain lead and should never be sipped from and bare hands in soil should be an obvious risk by now. The little toy rake that Molly's dad grabbed from the shed to make her feel as though she was participating in the yard work was cute, but on a recent recall list. Many plastic toys have unsafe levels of lead in the plastic, so paint is not always the culprit one has to watch for. On that note, remember Jennifer decorating the back deck with red balloons? Red dye and paint should be a flag as lead may be used in their manufacture, but in this case the balloons were not the problem. The chalky residue that the railing had begun to produce was. The problem was that she handled the railings and then went in to prepare food. Also if anyone were to have untied one of the helium filled balloons and handed it to a child during the party, the lead would be transferred from the railing to the children's hands.

The lead in the colored ink on the wrapping paper is a concern, although Molly did not play with it as she did last year. A little contact simply means a little lead, instead of a lot. And red wrapping paper? Risky.

The pewter cup is as dangerous a gift as the grandparents could have brought to the party because of its age. It was a bad move to let Molly drink punch out of it. The lesson: never put anything acidic in contact with a possible lead source. The pewter heirloom should go to the back of a high shelf of a closing cabinet, perhaps with a note slipped into it that says, "Don't drink out of me!"

The twins did not obtain any health benefit from their games of jacks. The jacks were the nice heavy ones that make for great playing, but they were heavy because they were weighted with lead. The sidewalk where they played with their lead jacks had been sprayed, as you recall, with a weed kill product that contained lead, as well as other carcinogenic agents that should never be used in anyone's backyard, especially where children or pets might go.

Molly's birthday scenario reminds us that the danger of lead can infiltrate life at any turn; its ability to put us at risk is ever-present. Yet, for parents of young children, it is easy to see how beginning to recognize high-risk lead sources is the most effective antidote available. As the hiding places of lead are revealed, you begin to see how the challenge of avoiding lead can be met head on for the benefit of those we care about most.

NOTES

CHAPTER 5

LEAD IN CHILDREN: NEGATIVE EFFECTS ON LEARNING AND THE CLASSROOM

Providing specialized educational services for children whose needs are unique or extraordinary is a daily challenge for our schools. When considering the resources, both monetary and human, involved in a mandate to include and support children with learning and behavioral challenges, it is easy to appreciate how the issue of lead-caused neurological damage impacts more than children and their families. As schools, struggle to teach a population showing up with more and more learning and behavior problems, the burden becomes society's responsibility and everyone's shared concern.

The resources needed to help lead babies succeed academically and socially at school are the focus of devoted teachers and their principals daily. What is not a part of their focus is the cause of the ever-increasing numbers of students with such problems. "What do we do?" overshadows concern or curiosity for *why* so many students arrive at school with learning disabled profiles, attention deficits, autism spectrum disorders diagnosis, or files thick with their "history of behavior." Despite how these teachers and classrooms are impacted, the educational community is not asking questions nor seeking out the research that has been on library shelves for as long a there have been schoolhouses.

Like schools, parents have not become champions of the cause of lead avoidance, an issue that government and science have been actively warning them about for decades. But there is a logical reason. The span of time between lead exposure and the detection of resulting brain dysfunction is long enough that any link between the cause and the effect is obscured. It is synonymous with being human that we do not react to that which does not cause us panic *right now.* We build houses in flood zones, fail to prepare for earthquakes that science promises are inevitable, and make light of our lack of self-control when we gorge on food that we know is clogging our arteries. We smoke.

Another factor that allows us to deny the connection between lead exposure and its damage is the reality that many teachers and parents believe that if a child just tried a little harder, if the school board just provided a little bit more support, everything would be better; the situation would improve; the disability would be overcome. If things were this simple, then lead damage would be an issue of far less urgency.

Equally disconcerting is that the disconnect between lead, the damage it causes and how our children are doing in school has perpetuated disbelief that the damage is even *real.* Many question the whole concept of what it means to have a learning disability or attention deficit, suggesting that perhaps it is simply the school system's excuse for why they have not been successful with the children they teach. To some, low IQ is the result of an under-stimulating home environment, problem behavior is lax parenting, and autism is an over-assigned label to something genetic. Given that the loss of human potential due to lead exposure is staggering, these explanations are convenient, but dangerously complacent. Understanding disability as the direct result of damage to the brain caused by exposure to lead is a pivotal point in the process of breaking the existing cycle. Familiarity with the magnitude and scope of its impact is also key.

Lead-Associated Reading Deficits in US Children
(Adapted from Lanphear BP, et al. Public Health Reports 2000; 115`521-529)

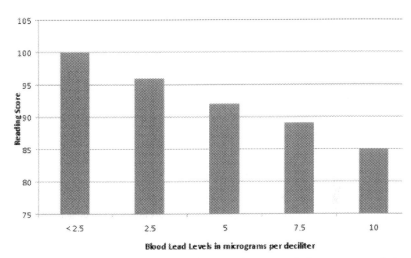

Lower level lead exposure decreases reading, math, non-verbal reasoning and short term memory scores in children.

Grade Four, Jackson Elementary

Marcus and his mother had managed to avoid the usual morning battle over what clothes to wear to school today. She had put out his clean clothes and Marcus had insisted on wearing yesterday's sweat pants and t-shirt. They were also the same sweat pants and t-shirt of the day before that, but she had decided not to notice, knowing there would be bigger battles to wage between now and boarding the school bus. Marcus, now eleven, allowed his mother to dress him while he watched as he twiddled his index finger against his thumb at eye level.

The bus pulled up in front of the house and its red stop sign eased down to halt passing cars. Marcus's mother kissed him good-bye, turned him back toward the bus, and guided him onboard. He would agree to be shown to his seat by the bus driver, belted in out of arm's-reach of anyone else, and then he would fixate on any windows that were down, insisting, by means of the noises that comprised his language, that they be closed. His mother dashed back up the walk and into the house.

Marcus's bus would stop a few minutes later and pick up other students from the class. At school an aide would be waiting for him and Mr. Wesley Hanover would be his teacher.

Seth, Joey and Andrea were students with their own unique struggles. Each morning they cheerfully boarded the bus in three quick stops following Marcus's. The sequence was etched in Marcus's brain and he would erupt if it were revised on a day when one of them was away. In the classroom, Andrea had a hard time staying focused; she could stay on task as long as the teacher stood next to her desk. But not Seth. He seemed to fall further behind with every week that passed; his spirit seemed to die a little more with each passing week and each dismal spelling test or math quiz he got back.

Last on the bus was Joey, usually running late with his jacket half off and his knapsack spilling things onto the sidewalk, despite that he was picked up a full thirty minutes later than the first students on the route. He was focused on everything all the time and he flitted from one thing to the next, and the next, and the next, making the others feel dizzy watching him. In the notes that Mr. Hanover had been left, he was told that Bill and Eric, along with Joey and Andrea were students with learning disabilities. This explained their slow progress, although it struck him as ironic that these students were entitled to leave the class each day for help with their reading, while students like Marcus with autism, or Seth with what Mr. Hanover learned was a mild intellectual disability, were left all day in the classroom with no specialized instruction.

But Wesley Hanover was assigned to Jackson Elementary only until a permanent grade four teacher could be hired. The year was already underway when the young teacher was asked to fill in and he was just happy as a substitute teacher that this assignment would last a while. So when Andrea and the other boys with the learning disabilities were interrupted in the middle of an important lesson, he was supportive and accommodating. He was even learning to be outwardly calm when Marcus jumped out of his seat and banged his head against the wall or the table, or grabbed the aide and hit her.

Despite the daily disruption and what sometimes seemed more like chaos than teaching, he worked hard to develop anchor activities to ensure that students had meaningful work suitable for their various ability levels and finish times. He created multiple versions of tests and assignments that would allow students to demonstrate their learning rather than penalize them for their weak skill sets, and designed activities and assignments that incorporated different levels of complexity in questioning and demands for abstract thinking. He tried to remember that various students preferred different learning modalities so his lessons were created to appeal to auditory, visual and kinesthetic learners. He had arrived anticipating that there would be a brief honeymoon period in which his presence and style would be a novelty, and for the most part he had seized this opportunity to make important connections and establish new routines.

Marcus was the exception. An unfamiliar person in the room had been enough to overwhelm him. And sure enough, Mr. Hanover had barely finished introducing himself and spelling H-A-N-O-V-E-R on the whiteboard when Marcus's rocking stopped, his chair flew out from under him and hit the wall, and a loud mournful yell accompanied a heavy-handed self-inflicted swack on the side of his own head.

In the split second that Mr. Hanover took to decide whether or not to get the class out of the room, the aide initiated moving Marcus to the hall. Twenty-seven drained looking faces first watched Marcus leave and then looked back at Mr. Hanover for their cue as to the next order of business.

Mr. Hanover quickly realized that his biggest allies in the classroom were the other students. Their wariness of Marcus was not unwarranted, but it added to a palpable tension that he decided early was not healthy. So during his first week at Jackson Elementary, Mr. Hanover spent one entire evening on his computer researching Autism Spectrum Disorders and another with Marcus's student file. At the back of Marcus's thick file, he had come across a therapist's report. The therapist had recommended a large ball as a way for Marcus to sit without rocking, but still meeting what she called his "vestibular needs." He had high hopes that it might not only provide a replacement for his rocking, but might also offset the boy's need to hit his own head. And she suggested a type of toy that might provide a bit of the tactile sensory diet that Marcus seemed to crave; he had seen something in the classroom cupboard that he now realized must be for Marcus. He made several other discoveries as he read through Marcus's file—that he was moderately mentally handicapped, and diagnosed with pica. He now understood why everything in Marcus's reach was eaten whether it was food or not.

In the morning, Mr. Hanover detoured to the gymnasium where he borrowed a large ball and then he retrieved that strange toy from the cupboard. He invited the class to pull their chairs and Marcus's ball into a large circle as the setting for the discussion he had planned. Marcus flew to the ball when he spotted it. He needed no instructions and balanced upon it for a full ten minutes before wandering off with his aide in close pursuit. It was a milestone, for Marcus rarely stayed in one place for longer than a minute. In his personal work corner at the back of the room, Marcus was sitting down, pulling and stretching the weird rubbery toy, but with a quiet concentration that made the teacher and the aide think that Marcus was actually listening to the class discussion. It seemed like progress.

In the circle discussion, Mr. Hanover was surprised to learn that the other students were not sure if they could catch what Marcus had. It was understandable that there were no friendly overtures toward him. Now that autism had been clarified, the class wanted to know why he could not talk and how they could communicate with him. Mr. Hanover was impressed and awakened by the earnest desire of what he had thought was a stressed classroom community. The children were willing to try to forge relationships with Marcus.

As the weeks passed, the calendar showed winter vacation drawing nearer. Mr. Hanover felt the struggle to maintain the students' focus intensify. In particular, the students with learning disabilities seemed to get frustrated quicker and be out of their seats constantly. During group work, there were conflicts and arguments between students who normally got along, and in general, the quality of work had tailed off. It seemed that almost every day, he was sending a behavior referral off to the office. He found himself starting to count down the days.

When the last trickle of students in the hallway was gone, Mr. Hanover sat at the desk he had become accustomed to calling his own. When he had come to fill in as a substitute, he was free to invest his energy how and where he wanted. Marcus had been a fascinating challenge that he had found hard to resist. He had a lot to be proud of in what he had accomplished in the short time he had been at Jackson Elementary. He stared out the window, thinking and watching the snow fall, despite the fact that the week was over and he was free to head off and start his winter holiday. In the moment, he had been thrilled to be told by the principal that he was staying on after the break until the end of the school year. But now the realization that this class was his responsibility had caught up with him.

He brought his gaze in from the cold and cued his attention on several empty desks that seemed to shout to him to notice them. They overflowed with papers and books, and readers and pencil boxes were strewn about. Joey's desk looked like he had left to go home in the middle of the last activity; Seth's looked like it had gotten hit by a car in the cross walk. Marcus's picture symbols were all in a jumble in his finished box and his schedule was empty. His FIRST and THEN card was pinned to the wall. It usually said FIRST: coat, THEN: bus. Today the picture symbols were: FIRST: bus, THEN: holiday. His uneaten, forgotten candy cane was pinned next to it.

A weary young Mr. Hanover wandered through the rows, sliding stray belongings into their respective desks for safekeeping. As he was about to turn off the lights and leave, he fought a sense of feeling overwhelmed by the prospect of six more months assigned to all of this need. Though little consolation, it occurred to him that this was probably how some of his students must feel—anxious and overwhelmed—every single day of their lives. At least, he could get out from under it for the next few weeks. They would have to take their disabilities home with them for vacation. And no one more than Marcus.

Jackson Elementary's grade four classroom setting provides insight into the realities that evolve as a result of early lead damage. And although we celebrate that there are bright, motivated teachers like Mr. Hanover who manage to cope, imagine the same classroom without the demands of autism, students struggling to grasp basic concepts, the inability to remember what was taught yesterday, or the need to re-teach what was missed when a student left the room for special help. We have a sense of the day-to-day classroom reality for students affected by lead. Now, what can science add to our perspective?

Scientific researchers have studied the brain in a number of ways over the past few decades to demonstrate once and for all that there are physical differences in the brains of lead-affected individuals.

For instance, there are specific measurable differences in those who have been identified as having a learning disability. While science has always had autopsy as a research tool, its limitations are obvious. The CT (Computed Tomography) scan, the MRI (Magnetic Resonance Imaging), the EEG (Electroencephalogram), the PET (Positron Emission Tomography) scan, and the SPECT (Single Photon Emission Computed Tomography) scan are tools that have allowed us to look inside to watch and measure the differences in people's brains.

One of the most pronounced differences between a typical brain and the brain of an individual who tests as having a learning disability is that the learning disabled brain does not share the asymmetry of the typical brain. For example, the temporal lobe located in the left hemisphere of the brain, a part of the brain activated during reading activities, is larger than the temporal lobe in the right hemisphere in typical readers. This is not the case in the brains of individuals with reading-related learning disabilities.[42] In addition to the discovery that asymmetry related to brain size in key structures of the brain is related to learning disability, differences in how the brain works have also been documented with the help of modern medical technology.

Functional neuroimaging techniques allow us to measure brain activity while subjects are engaged in a task such as reading. An MRI is a non-invasive method that measures blood flow, while PET and SPECT methods involve the injection of radioactive materials. SPECT scan results have indicated that subjects with learning disabilities show under-functioning in the occipital lobe while reading in comparison to subjects without learning disabilities. Employing the EEG, research has shown that subjects with learning disabilities produced less electrical activity in the parietal lobe, in comparison to subjects without learning disabilities.[43]

Individuals who have received assessments and subsequently have been diagnosed with autism show some other important physical characteristics that confirm the relationship between lead exposure and these brain differences. Teeth, like bone, are important biological markers linking prenatal and newborn lead exposure to a sequence of heavy metal exposure that will be explored in detail in chapter seven. At the very least, the knowledge of which part of the brain is required for which function, referenced against critical times of development and vulnerability to interference, allows us to enhance our understanding and avoid repeating our past mistakes. The schedule of embryonic and fetal development from chapter two does not identify lead sources; however, it can offer insight into lead exposure timeframes for students like Joey, Seth, Andrea or Marcus. We can deduce that exposure occurred in all pregnancies between weeks three and twenty when the main development of their central nervous systems occurred. If we had access to their baby teeth, which would reveal lead levels when tested, we could narrow the window of lead exposure to a six-week period, from six and a half weeks to week twelve, since we know exactly when teeth are formed in utero.

Difficulty with reading, writing, attention and social relationships does not, in and of itself, indicate evidence of brain damage. Certainly the ability to do a great many of the tasks that life, and school in particular, demand is impeded or impacted by whether or not the tasks have been properly or adequately taught. Even cultural context and lack of relevant experiences to draw on can play a role in a child's ability to excel or lag behind typically developing peers. Some inabilities related to learning and behavior, though, *are* neurologically based.

Whether difficulty is encountered with reading, writing, math concepts, listening, speaking or concentrating depends on the sequence of toxin exposure to the brain and obvious variables such as timing, combined effect with other neurotoxins and the amount of toxin exposure. Although a specific, measurable causal link between lead and learning is difficult to track, a school-age child's inability to rhyme words, learn the alphabet, or notice when words start with the same sound are early signs that the brain is not functioning as it should. And these are precisely the sorts of skills that the brain struggles with when it has been compromised by lead during its early development.

Who amongst us would intentionally or knowingly sentence a child to a life of frustration at being behind academically in school, being unable to read or write, or to experience the emotional pain of not fitting in socially? It is uncomfortable to consider lead exposure as a life sentence of compromised potential, but it is just that. With science able to demystify what children, their teachers and their parents experience as the human side of the irreversible fallout of early lead exposure, there is nothing left to hide behind. In the chapters ahead, the knowledge needed to prevent the cycle from repeating will be set into motion with the tools to make prevention a reality.

NOTES

CHAPTER 6

LEAD AND TEENS:
IMPACT ON IQ AND BEHAVIOR

How can the wide discrepancy in crime rates between cities across Canada and the United States—for that matter around the world—be explained? The fact that the number of toxic metal releases in a given area of population correlates closely with the amount of violent crime offers an important clue.

Even though causation in behavioral issues is almost invariably multifactorial, antisocial behavior, like cognitive function, has been associated with neurotoxic exposure for much of the twentieth century. Mounting evidence has been amassed over recent decades from the fields of behavior, neuropsychology and biology that confirms that the brain dysfunction caused by early, low-level exposure to lead results in the specific brain dysfunction that is associated with the behavior we find with ADHD, delinquency and violence.

The change in understanding between what was previously accepted and what is now known is in the area of exposure threshold for damage. It was previously assumed that only high levels of exposure caused damage and regulations were set accordingly. The more recent realization that neurotoxic effects occur at even the lowest levels of exposure, and that they can occur before a baby is born, has offered new, if not shocking insight into a long list of trends related to behavior, including school drop-out, delinquency, drug use and violent crime.

One of these well-noted trends is the difference between crime rates in rural and urban areas. The US Bureau of Justice Statistics, for example, reports that "central cities, particularly those with populations between 250,000 and 499,999, have the highest per capita rates of violent crime."[44] When in 1999 homicide rates fell for the first time in three decades, with the bigger declines in busy, urban areas, the Bureau of Justice Statistics explained that it was related to the prevalence of guns. There is significant evidence to suggest otherwise. As leaded gasoline was phased out around the country, blood lead levels, particularly in busy urban centers, dropped, not surprisingly.[45]

Lead and Violent Crime

Another trend that warrants examination is the relationship between documented brain abnormalities and the population who occupy North America's extensive system of prisons. Many prison inmates have records of learning disabilities and histories of poor success in school, already suggestive of prenatal or infant lead exposure. But not *all* individuals with learning challenges indulge in the kinds of activities and behavior that land them in prison, so mindfulness of sweeping inferences is imperative.

However, through the use of magnetic resonance imaging, MRI, researchers identified that the reduction in the amount of prefrontal gray matter—a loss of brain neurons observable in the brains of lead-exposed children—is the same in adults with antisocial personality disorder such as is common in prison populations. The tendency to be "deceitful, reckless, impulsive, irresponsible and lacking in remorse and empathy" is symptomatic of a toxic brain injury, despite the fact that many are heavily invested in the theory that poverty, poor parenting, or negative social influences are to blame.[46] On the contrary, the research is overwhelming that prenatal or early childhood damage to the prefrontal cortex of the brain is a critical influence in violent criminal and anti-social behavior.[47]

In a study published in the May 2000 *Environmental Research Journal*, Rick Nevin performed a statistical analysis of childhood lead exposure and violent crime rates and unwed pregnancies.[48] Nevin produced two very significant findings, both of which deserve careful attention. First, he analyzed statistics on rates of murder, rape, robbery, and aggravated assault within various geographical communities. He revealed that childhood lead exposure was such a key factor in violent crime that it explained eighty-eight percent of the increase in violent crime that was recorded between 1960 and 1996. Equally noteworthy, Nevin showed that ninety percent of the increased rate of unwed pregnancy (abortion and unwed births) for women age fifteen to nineteen was linked to childhood lead exposure.[49]

The damage that lead causes to the frontal lobes of the developing brain results in a lifelong loss of control over aggressive urges and impulsivity. At a very basic level, this knowledge forces us to rethink what we believe about delinquent behavior and crime as well as how society should act and organize itself in response. Understanding that delinquent and antisocial behavior are products of early childhood lead exposure is an astounding realization but long overdue.

Lead and African Americans

As we unpack our perceptions about people and why they do what they do, long-held beliefs and understandings must be set aside. For instance, why is there a disproportionate representation of high school drop-outs, prisoners and the poor amongst African Americans? Research on lead absorption highlights calcium deficiency as a critical factor in lead susceptibility, leaving those who are lactose intolerant significantly more vulnerable. Lactose intolerance, relative to the population in general, is more common—extremely common in fact—in those of African descent. In the US, eighty-six percent of African Americans get less than half the daily recommended amount of calcium.[50] When the US National Medical Association studied this trend, they determined that while taste and cultural preference were factors, avoidance was largely due to lactose intolerance.[51]

The estimated prevalence of lactose maldigestion (or lactase non-persistence) varies among different ethnic and racial groups in the U.S. Among Asian Americans, African Americans, Native American Indians, and Hispanics, an estimated 50% to 100% are reported to be lactose maldigesters, compared to 15% of Caucasians.[52]

The relationship between lead and crime has a new and revealing significance when applied to populations with a biological predisposition to absorb lead. Not only are they more likely to have a lead-caused learning disability, they are also statistically more prone to lead-caused frontal lobe damage which as we know is related to behavior.

Lead and Video Games

Another twist is in our widely held assumptions about violent video games and the impact they are having on our youth. There is considerable controversy over the influence that the virtual violence of video games has on current societal trends. It is a defensible argument that not everyone becomes aggressive after exposure to video games, yet there is plenty of research to show that some people do. One study showed that adolescents who play violent video games for extended periods of time, (more than thirteen hours a week) "tend to be more aggressive, are more prone to confrontation with their teachers, may engage in fights with their peers and see a decline in school achievement."[53]

This same study also saw a decrease in helping behaviors associated with these individuals. Furthering the evidence, researchers from the Indiana School of Medicine used magnetic resonance technology to monitor brain activity as teens watched and played violent video games. The researchers observed activity in the amygdala, the region of the brain involved in emotional arousal and which activates the anger center. The part of the brain connected to the ability to focus, concentrate and exercise self-control showed less activity, thereby potentially slowing brain development.[54]

Accordingly, those children who have suffered early damage to this same portion of their brain that suppresses aggression and regulates self control are left vulnerable to the effects of exposure to violence. They are *lead babies* who live out the legacy of damaged inhibition mechanisms as teenagers and adults, more likely to act out the aggression they experience in the game world. They are less able to regulate the urges of aggression that come about as video game violence intensely stimulates key parts of the brain.

Lead and Trauma

Similarly, we see differences in the ways people cope with severe trauma, some individuals developing post-traumatic stress disorder, while others carry on seemingly emotionally intact.[55] Tamara Gurvits and colleagues studied a group of subjects who had survived traumatic experiences. Some were sexually abused as children, while others had served and returned from the Vietnam War. When neurological and psychological tests were done, researchers found that "subjects with Post Traumatic Stress Syndrome reported more neurodevelopmental problems and more childhood attention deficit hyperactivity disorder symptoms and had lower IQs, all of which were significantly correlated with neurologic soft signs."[56] Individuals with neurological deficits, such as those caused by lead damage, are more apt to suffer post traumatic stress symptoms and cope with traumatic stress less effectively.

Lead and Addiction

Studies involving the biology and chemistry of addiction are uncovering new implications that point back to early, low-level lead exposure. As mentioned previously, early and in utero lead exposure, even at very low doses, is known to cause damage to the prefrontal lobes. Research confirms that frontal lobe dysfunction is a risk factor and important predictor for alcohol abuse. Even slight impairment to cognitive ability and language skills has been shown to increase risk for drug and alcohol abuse.

Ralph Tarter and colleagues studied girls and substance abuse. They found that compared to controls, girls with substance abuse problems were "impaired on cognitive tests measuring verbal intelligence, attention, perceptual efficiency, language competence, and educational achievement."[57] There is also evidence that some drug addiction is actually a self-medication of the symptoms that individuals with ADHD suffer.

In a study by the US National Institute on Drug Abuse, adult cocaine abusers reported to researchers that they first started using cocaine as a way of self-medicating symptoms of ADHD, namely, difficulties in paying attention, keeping still and suppressing impulsive behaviors.[58] In either scenario, the pathway to addiction traces back to the damage that lead caused during early brain development.

Misunderstanding Scott: Delinquent or Victim

The seven-minute warning bell calling the kids back from their midday lunch break sang out loudly, both inside and outside the school building. A group in the smoke pit, a dirt patch adjacent to the school property under a large fir tree that offered protection on rainy days, scattered as a vice principal approached. Most students funneled through the front and side doors of the huge box of a building, while a few picked up their pace as they returned from the snack bar at the service station on the corner.

Scott still had a lit cigarette dangling from his mouth as he crossed the school parking lot, heading away from the school. When he reached the sidewalk in front of the school he looked in both directions before deciding. He did not have a destination in mind yet, but why would he walk up a hill when he could walk down? Either way, he had had enough of school for one day. He had gone to two classes, even though he had arrived to Social Studies twenty-five minutes late. But Ms. Johnston hadn't even noticed him come in and she didn't seem to notice that Scott had left part way through the block either.

The truth was, Ms. Johnson was more than a little aware of when Scott was in her class and when he wasn't. As he came and went, the class dynamic changed as though it were wired to an on/off switch. The class carried on when Scott would saunter in but they sensed that a confrontation may ensue.

Beth Johnson might be at the laissez-faire end of the teacher style spectrum but she was no pushover. She was a veteran teacher who knew when to make a point and when to listen to the hairs on the back of her neck. And when to read every page of a student file. She was well informed of Scott's propensity to escalate if confronted in front of his peers. She and a couple of colleagues had discussed Scott in the staffroom over lunch one day and decided there was nothing to be gained by engaging in what was clearly an invitation to a power struggle.

Johnson's Social Studies class was a waste of time, but nothing compared to Turnbull's resource room block. To Scott there was stupid, and then there was humiliating. He'd been in special classes for social development all through grade school and now he was stuck going to resource room.

Scott shunned the other students even though deep, deep down, he knew that his ability was even lower than some of theirs. Scott's cognitive ability was indeed in a range considered as a mild intellectual disability, a few points south of seventy, low enough to qualify him for special education services. Academically, he was slow to learn new things and years behind his peers in reading and math.

He railed against this offer of help by making sure he did not bring any books or anything to write with. But Mrs. Turnbull never ceased to amaze him with a bottomless supply of new pencils. When she saw that he had come without, she simply handed him one. He would return the favor by chomping teeth marks into them and wearing the erasers down to stubs.

Shop class was different. Scott liked and looked forward to it. Sometimes there were too many instructions at once and he got that panicky feeling in his stomach. But Mr. Swensen seemed to always know when to show up at Scott's side to give him a bit of a hand and get him back on track. He was getting good at oil changes and tire patching. But he liked bigger jobs that meant taking engines apart. As a steady stream of junkers came in for repair, Mr. Swensen would show him exactly what needed to be done to remove an old dead battery or free up a leaky radiator.

But there was no shop class in the rotation on Thursdays, so there was nothing left to hold Scott's interest or to draw him back to school now that lunch was done. As a few clusters of students passed him, they stepped around him, making sure that in their rush to get back before the final bell, they did not accidentally bump shoulders with him. They stepped widely around him and did not speak or make eye contact. Good, he thought. You'd better watch out. Every kid at Senator Secondary knew that Scott Westwold had "issues."

As the end of the sidewalk approached, Scott threw down the stub of his cigarette and jaywalked across four lanes of traffic. The crosswalk, with its chirping noises and its juvenile Walk / Don't Walk signals was too much like conformity. A car slowed in realization that he was taking his time crossing and Scott liked that. He made a decision to head over to the bus loop where he was sure to meet up with someone he knew who was skipping from somewhere, and then he reached into his jean jacket breast pocket and produced a tightly rolled joint. He passed it by his lips to dampen the paper slightly, lit it with a silver skull-shaped lighter, and proceeded to smoke it defiantly in the open as he walked and thought about what else he could do to dull the angst in the pit of his stomach.

Part of what drew Scott to the bus loop, besides knowing he'd find some other truant who was willing to hang out for a few hours, was the Gun and Tackle Shop and the Dollar Store next door. He regularly helped himself to penny candy, casually stuffing it in his pockets when no one was looking. He didn't steal from the Gun and Tackle Shop since the owner never let him past the doorway. But there was lots to look at in the window that reminded him of the times he used to go fishing in the summer. He used to have his own rod and tackle box, and he knew which leader was for what kind of fishing, and how much weight he would need depending on how deep the fish were. And the guns were cool too. He had a particular fascination with guns, though not quite the respect his father was trying to teach him. But he knew a lot about handling them and firing them as this was something he used to do often with his dad on a Saturday at the firing range.

With the bus loop in view now, he looked for a recognizable silhouette, a familiar face. A group of three boys stood smoking against a cement planter that apparently doubled as a garbage can judging by the trash that was strewn in with the greenery. He knew one of the boys so he wandered over nonchalantly to test the waters of whether he might be welcome. He adjusted the thick silver chain around his neck, something he'd bullied off of a kid in the summer. It was a trophy for sure and he wore it like a confidence charm.

He was glad he had remembered it today because he hated not being smart. And he hated the hyper feeling that he got when he had to think too hard or sit too long. He knew that the price a guy had to pay to have friends was to go along with whatever they said. Oh, and to be tough, and never let them know he wasn't smart. Scott had a plan in his head. Better to make them think you were such a bad ass that they kicked you out of school than to have them find out you weren't smart enough to pass.

A remarkable amount is known about how and when brain damage is sustained through infancy and childhood as an outcome of lead exposure. Yet for a young man like Scott, struggling in both the cognitive and the behavioral domains, the reasons for his failure to learn like his peers, or for his oppositional disposition, escape his teachers, his friends and his family. The shift in understanding the role of lead in IQ and behavior cannot come too soon for Scott to have a happy and fulfilled life.

We know when damage to the brain related to cognitive ability and brain function related to reading, math and learning in general has occurred. A loss of spatial working memory (things we do in our head without talking) and attention flexibility (how easily we can move our focus from one thing to another) cue us that the brain is not functioning optimally.

Scott's below average intelligence is not a product of a faulty genetic combination, poor parenting or a medical accident during his delivery as a baby—at least not in isolation. Scott's IQ is below seventy and falling because as his brain was forming, between conception and sometime in week sixteen of his mother's pregnancy, lead was either leaching out of her bones and transferring to him, or his mother was being exposed to new sources. And therefore Scott was too. Scott's cognitive abilities continue to decline as he keeps on handling lead acid batteries and worn-out car radiators. As long as he is exposed to these high-risk lead sources, he will be a steady conduit of lead via his skin, hair, shoes and clothes, in the home where he lives, increasing the risk to himself and his family.

But the auto mechanics shop is not the only source of lead at school. There are many, from the water fountains in the hallway to the hot chocolate machine in the cafeteria. Ironically, though, it is the pencils in the resource room that contain the lead that is a daily problem for Scott. It is a myth that pencils were once made with lead and are now made with graphite. In fact, pencils have never contained lead as their writing material. But Mrs. Turnbull goes through volumes of pencils in the resource room and orders boxes of cheap pencils to save her department money. It is the lead-containing yellow paint on the pencils that has snuck by the retailer and is ending up in contact with students' hands and making its way to their mouths as pencils inevitably seem to do.

The impulsivity and inability to concentrate that Scott has battled since faced with school tasks as early as kindergarten is dulled by the marijuana he smokes. The cannabis provides effective relief to a large subset of smokers like Scott who are essentially self-medicating the discomfort of being ADHD and trying to learn to cope.

Scott seems to have a taste for all things lead. As a boy, Scott handled pure lead each time he opened his tackle box and tied a weight onto his fishing line. Time spent at the firing range would entail ingesting airborne lead dust and breathing in vapor, possibly the worst way to bring lead from the environment into the human system. That this was a pastime of his father's as well suggests that his father might have been bringing lead into the house regularly, even if he had not taken his son along. The metal in his cheap, imported lighter is a small but frequent source of exposure as he handles it hourly. The penny candy that Scott steals and eats is imported from Mexico, where laws are lax and lead is often contained in candy. Each of these lead exposures is in itself a relatively minute amount of lead particulate. However, strung across weeks and years of Scott's life, the cumulative intake is plainly visible in an X-ray of his bones. It is no coincidence that bone lead levels in delinquent teens are significantly higher than their regular peers. Not just a little higher, but, as tibia bone x-rays showed in a study in 2002, on average, eleven times higher.[59] This comes as little surprise, as there are two well-documented correlating factors with criminal activity; lead toxicity and anemia. Anemia, as any doctor can tell you, is a symptom of lead toxicity.

Scott's story of frustration and anger is made all the more disturbing by the fact that his difficulties have environmental origins that could have been avoided. Furthermore, the discouragement and misbehavior that students like Scott present extend far beyond schools. While we cannot say what the future holds for Scott and thousands just like him, "the best predictor for juvenile delinquency and eventual criminal violence is the degree of lead poisoning" found in children at age seven.[60]

Scott is not the result of bad parenting, a low socioeconomic status or bad traits genetically inherited. Once exposed to lead, the brain circuitry that allows for the ability to regulate behavior and emotions is damaged. The damage is permanent.

Lead concentrates in growing bones as shown in these radiographs of a child's knees and hands. The white metaphyseal are referred to as 'lead lines.'

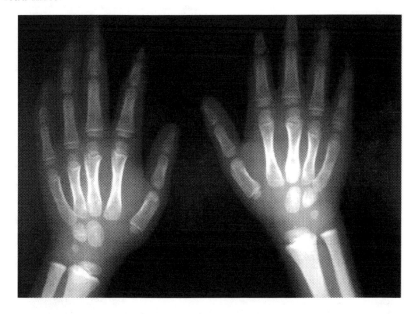

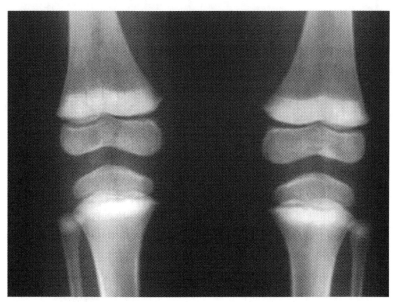

Photos courtesy of Dr. Celsa Lopez, Clinical Epidemiological Research Unit. IMSS, Torreon, Mexico

Lead and the Biology of the Brain

What specifically does lead do to the unborn or newly born brain? The damage occurs in the neocortex, the part of the brain that processes information. The neo-cortex contains some one hundred billion cells, each with one thousand to ten thousand synapses (connections), and has roughly one hundred million meters of wiring all packaged into a structure that, if we were able to un-crumple it and lay it out flat, would equal the size of a dinner napkin.[61] The internal structure of the neo-cortex is stacked layers of cells, organized into columns that will do the job of what is referred to as "sensory mapping" shortly after birth. Lead's interference with certain cell receptors that should later be responsible for spurring on that vital sensory mapping activity, is critical.

Instead of the brain's nerve cells, the dendrites, growing and spreading like tree branches, they will be stunted and their ability to send out signals reduced.[62] The cell receptors whose job it is to trigger this flurry of new growth are damaged and no such message is received by the awaiting nerve cells.

The fact that research has shown that damage to the developing neo-cortex increases with increased exposure to lead in utero is important to consider when the lead and behavior connection moves beyond ADHD and behavior disorders to link with delinquency and drug abuse. There is no room for doubt that diminished growth of neuron clusters resulting in stunted sensory mapping is a direct cause of the inability to concentrate, hyperactivity and anti-social behavior that is growing exponentially in our schools and becoming criminal behavior and drug addiction in our streets.[63]

Ignoring the fact that behavior is an outcome of physical changes to the brain caused by heavy metals and other neurotoxins is simply not an option when science confirms that lead alone accounts for eleven to thirty-nine percent of arrested delinquents.[64] The issue of lead exposure demands serious attention *now* if the trends in crime and delinquency are to be turned around for the benefit of the upcoming generation. The long-term consequences of prenatal exposure to lead are dire.

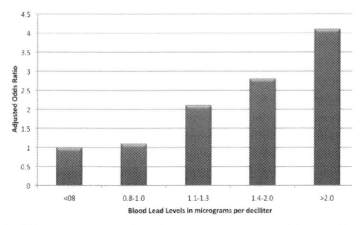

Risk of ADHD by Blood Lead Concentration in US Children, 4 to 15 years, NHANES 1992-2002

Adapted from Braun, J. et al. EHP 2006;17:500-505

The risk of ADHD increases with lead exposure as measured in blood lead levels.

Lowered Intelligence in the Lead-Exposed Brain

Lead-caused brain damage and potential lifelong impairment to cognitive ability which manifests itself as ADHD, learning disabilities or anti-social behavior are an urgent concern. However, the implications for intelligence are equally concerning. Here is where the issue of exposure takes us beyond the threshold of the infant and the brain in its early stages of development. Ongoing lead exposure throughout one's life has the unfortunate effect of diminishing one's intelligence. Therefore, lead exposure concerns us all.

Researchers report that blood lead levels (even though readings of lead levels in blood do not reflect stored lead levels in brain tissue and bone), well below the level currently defined as toxic in children (ten micrograms per deciliter) are associated with poorer cognitive skills. A research team at the Children's Hospital Medical Center in Cincinnati evaluated data for 4,853 American children between the ages of six and sixteen. They found that as blood lead levels rise, starting at concentrations as low as 2.5 micrograms per deciliter, scores for reading, math and other basic skills significantly drop. This relationship is independent of race, region of the country, parental education and other socioeconomic factors.[65]

The lack of understanding that underpins the average person's nonchalant attitude toward lead is paralleled by an under-reaction to estimates of IQ reduction being mentioned during discussions about the impact of lead. Most people do not know their own IQ, and probably would not know if a five-point decline in IQ was a little or a lot.

Five points is a lot, relatively speaking. Predictions of IQ loss in North America due to lead exposure in children and adults are in the range of four IQ points, nationwide, for the initial quantities of lead that enter the body and become stored. Levels of blood lead up to ten micrograms per deciliter would lower IQ by seven points. And levels over ten micrograms per deciliter would drop IQ by another two points. Note that it is the first few micrograms of lead that do the most damage to cognitive potential.

So what does a five-, six-, seven-point difference in IQ mean in terms of personal potential? In school achievement, it could mean the difference between an A or a B—getting into the university of choice, or settling for a second or third choice—maybe attending a community college. At the other end of the scale, it could mean the difference between a low C average and failing; this could literally mean the difference between staying in school and dropping out. For those already at the low end of average, a seventy IQ indicates mental retardation. When we translate these differences into educational opportunity and earning potential, small numbers take on big significance. Each IQ point lost is potentially a lost opportunity in the increased competition that exists in a global economy, or an increased cost to society by requiring special education services in school and financial and community support as adults. In the workplace, intellectual impairment and even mild loss of function translate silently into increased rates of workplace injury.

The numbers of students who will require special education services in North American schools is projected to double in the next decade. This fact alone will change how schools go about the business of education and what the quality of education for students along the intelligence continuum looks like.

A 1995 attempt to quantify the combined costs of lost cognitive ability and associated behavioral outcomes estimated seven billion dollars in earnings per each microgram per deciliter of lead.[66] But consider the cost of removal. The latest figures on fully removing lead from our environment would come at an estimated cost of eight thousand dollars per saved IQ point. It has already been argued in boardrooms around conference tables that it is not worth the cost.[67]

NOTES

CHAPTER 7

POTENTIATION:
THE MISSING PIECE OF THE AUTISM
PUZZLE

Many have had the experience of taking a prescription drug and having a glass or two of wine at dinner only to find themselves "under the table." They have experienced what is known in science labs as potentiation. Pharmacologically, potentiation is when the synergistic action of two drugs is greater than the sum of the effects of each when taken on its own. A person becomes a slurring drunk after drinking what they normally tolerate. On any other day, the same dose of the prescription does not make them drowsy or slow their reactions. Mixing the two substances, they need to find a designated driver and go home to bed.

In some medical scenarios, drugs are administered in combination specifically for the potentiation effect. In cancer treatment, for example, insulin has been administered to patients because the presence of insulin boosts the effect of some cancer drugs. In the worlds of alchemy and neurotoxicology, potentiation or synergistic effect, as it is also referred to, occurs in exactly the same way. Heavy metals such as lead and mercury have a tendency to potentiate with one another just as the pharmaceuticals do. Too often, research on lead and mercury is done separately and their tendency to potentiate is overlooked.

As early as 1978, a study of rats found that where lead was present, the toxic effect of mercury increased to at least one hundred times what it is alone. Regardless of the fact that potentiation has been established, most toxicology tests today continue to be conducted on single metals. This is highly problematic and is blocking progress towards a widespread understanding of the role of heavy metals in autism.

Potentiation is not limited to heavy metals that exist in nature or in the body. Testosterone intensifies the toxic impact of heavy metal through potentiation, a critical fact when unraveling the mystery of why autism, learning disabilities and ADHD so predominantly affect boys. For instance, the incidence of autism amongst boys is ten times that of girls.[68] Testosterone potentiates the toxicity of mercury, while estrogen has been shown to have protective properties. Researchers report that the severity of autism correlates with levels of testosterone in prenatal amniotic fluid and that a considerable percentage of autistic children show elevated plasma testosterone levels.[69]

Potentiation, above all else, may ultimately be the key that unlocks the mystery of an increase in the prevalence of autism that has taken off since the early 1980s on every continent in the world; an 805 percent increase in the United States since 1992.[70] Mercury, the second most toxic substance known to man behind only deadly plutonium, is making its way to the developing brains of babies, both born and in utero, in a way that parallels the saga of lead. When it arrives, however, its usual terrible toxic impact is magnified wildly in those children in whom lead toxicity is already a serious factor.

Several studies report that individuals with autism have higher blood lead levels concentrations and that high lead levels may contribute to either the onset or acceleration of the development of the symptoms of autism.[71] For example, researchers from the Knights of Columbus Research Center reviewed six cases of inner city children who were diagnosed with infantile autism and lead toxicity. It was concluded that in at least two cases the lead may have contributed to the onset or acceleration of autism.[72] Another study that compared mean blood lead levels of eighteen children with autism with that of sixteen children who did not have autism showed that blood lead level concentration was notably higher in children who were diagnosed with autism. Forty-four percent of children who had autism had blood lead levels greater than two standard deviations above the mean for children without autism.[73]

A study published in the *Journal of Applied Research,* examined case histories of two severely lead-exposed children who subsequently developed autism or autistic symptoms. Based on their findings, the research emphasized that environmental factors, such as lead exposure, play a definite role in the etiology of autism. The authors of the study explain,

> The ability of lead poisoning to induce symptoms of autism is also relevant to cases of preexisting pervasive developmental disorders irrespective of etiology. Such individuals have a greater propensity to engage in pica, and as a result, are more likely to become lead poisoned. In such cases, lead poisoning can be expected not only to negatively impact neurocognitive functioning, but also to potentially exacerbate the preexisting symptoms of autism.[74]

A review covering the years from 1987 to 1992 compared a group of seventeen children diagnosed with autism and treated for lead exposure with a randomly selected group of thirty children without autism, but who were also treated for lead exposure. Compared to the control group, children with autism had elevated blood lead levels for longer periods and despite close monitoring and environmental improvements, seventy-five percent were subsequently re-exposed.

Additionally, authors of manuals on identifying and treating autism advise that children suspected of having autism need to be tested for blood lead levels. Consider just one example:

> From research suggesting that individuals with autism have higher blood-lead concentrations, and the hypothesis that lead poisoning may contribute to

the onset or acceleration of the development of ASD symptoms, lead screening is recommended for all children referred for an autism screening.[75]

So far, research on the cause of autism, has been narrowly focused on several competing theories. Even the identification of mercury as the causal agent, has so far resulted in inconclusive controversy. Potentiation, however, sheds important new light on the cause of autism and how both lead and mercury are involved. It is no wonder that the current practice of looking for a single cause of autism has not produced results that allow us to avoid the things that cause it.

Would it be outrageous to suppose that when lead potentiates with mercury in the system of a child, the effect is autism? The degree of impairment and the period of onset may be related to all of the variables that logically now come into play: the amount of neurotoxic exposure and the stage of development that the brain was at when the exposure occurred.

The Life of Mercury

The fact that lead synergistically affects the already deadly toxicity of mercury does not bode well for the situation in our streams and lakes. Lead sinkers and other fishing related paraphernalia are widespread and they are the focus of a campaign to phase them out and quickly ban them completely in some US states. While the death by lead poisoning of waterfowl and birds of prey that ingest lead tackle or eat fish that have done so is concerning, (it is estimated that a single lead sinker could kill a loon) the problem of lead left behind by anglers is made more sinister by the potentiation effect where mercury is present too.

The environmental persistence of metals such as lead and mercury only adds to the problem. Once they are mined and introduced into the food chain, they are here to stay. Once they travel through the environment or food chain and end up inside us, they are essentially ours for life. Or death, depending on what kind of cocktail we have inherited, ingested or inhaled. Volumes of evidence suggest that interactions and combinations of metals in the body are critical catalysts for life-altering brain damage, as well as the formation of cancers and other diseases.

Organic mercury compounds, such as methylmercury, are formed when mercury combines with carbon. Microscopic organisms convert inorganic mercury into methylmercury, which is the most common organic mercury compound found in the environment. Methylmercury accumulates up the food chain by varied pathways.

Volcanic eruptions significantly contribute to the amount of mercury found in the atmosphere. Modern day industry, specifically coal and gas-fired power plants, gold mining operations, industrial processes such as chlorine production, smelting and manufacturing continue to introduce dangerous levels of mercury into the environment.

Products containing mercury are ending up in incinerators and landfills and recycling back into the environment. As a result, mercury is readily making its way into the human food supply. Because so much lead and mercury end up in oceans, lakes and streams, seafood has become extensively contaminated and is a major source of mercury to humans.

Other highly problematic sources of mercury exist. Pharmaceutical products such as vaccines and dental amalgam expose humans, both children and adults, to mercury.

The toxicity of mercury to the central nervous system has been extensively demonstrated and documented. One does not have to look any further than Japan's Minamata disaster of 1952, when Japan's Chisson Chemical Company dumped mercury into Minamata Bay. When surrounding residents ate the contaminated fish, widespread mercury poisoning occurred. Amongst the nearly four hundred affected people, sixty-eight died. Of those, twenty-two were unborn children. Again in Japan, in 1965 in Niigata, 330 people ate contaminated fish and either became ill with mercury poisoning or died after a factory dumped large amounts of mercury in a river. Follow-up studies revealed an increase in autism rates in the area in the years after the 1965 spill.[76] In Iraq in 1961, in Pakistan in 1963 and in Guatemala in 1966, large numbers of people were harmed by eating flour made from seeds treated with mercury-containing fungicides.[77]

Household Mercury Sources

There are many household and everyday mercury sources, ranging from common name brand household cleansers to greeting cards. It is important to be aware of them to avoid accidental exposure and to dispose of them in ways that do not add to the existing environmental load. Elemental or metallic mercury is the liquid metal used in thermometers, button cell batteries, electrical switches, and household cleaning products. Enclosed in glass or metal and left undisturbed, vapors are contained and not a direct risk. But uncontained room temperature mercury can evaporate and become an invisible, odorless toxic vapor that is extremely dangerous in poorly ventilated areas. Inorganic compounds and organic compounds such as phenylmercury acetate and ethylmercury, commonly taking the form of white powders or crystals, have been commonly used as fungicides, antiseptics and disinfectants. While what was widespread use has been mostly discontinued, small amounts continue to be used legally in pharmaceuticals, both in prescription and over-the-counter products.

The Vaccine Controversy

In the 1930s, the pharmaceutical company, Eli Lilly, developed a vaccine preservative called Thimerosal. Containing 49.5 percent mercury, the preservative was used in vaccines and other health products.

Concern arose when mercury-based preservatives were linked to the depletion of the protective anti-oxidant, glutathione. Without glutathione, the body is unable to rid itself of the neurotoxin mercury. Individuals diagnosed with autism have in common both low levels of glutathione and poor ability to eliminate mercury. Shortly after the mercury preservative was introduced into vaccines, reports of children with autism appeared in the medical literature.

In 1943, the first paper to identify children with autism was published by American psychologist, Leo Kanner. He had been observing autistic behavior in children beginning in the 1930s, eventually giving it the label of "early infantile autism." Although unaware of Kanner's work, an Austrian by the name of Hans Asperger published "Autistic Psychopathology in Childhood" just one year later. While Kanner did not specifically estimate the incidence of autism at the time, he did believe it to be extremely rare. Twenty years later, however, the first results of an epidemiological study of children with the behavior pattern described by Kanner were published by Victor Lotter. A prevalence rate of 4.5 per ten thousand children was established for Middlesex, England.[78]

In 1948, it was realized that a cluster of symptoms in babies known as Pink Disease was in fact mercury poisoning. Mercury was immediately withdrawn from baby products such as teething powders and the incidence of Pink Disease was all but eliminated.[79]

When babies are born in hospitals, one of the first things that they receive is routine eye drops. Ophthalmic solutions commonly contain mercury based preservative. Newborns who were not exposed to mercury in utero may get their first exposure in the delivery room. Furthermore, newborns will have inherited some level of mercury from the fish their mother ate, the amalgam in their mother's teeth, the mercury-containing flu shot their mother may have had, or the cosmetics that she wore.

The amount of lead that has transferred from the mother's bones and bloodstream to the developing fetus, added to the amount of in utero mercury or other toxic exposure that has already occurred, may in fact be the variable that accounts for the spectrum of autism incidence, ranging from no evidence of autism to cases that are extremely severe.

Also at birth, babies are routinely given a Hepatitis B vaccine. By the time a North American infant has left the hospital, he or she has run the risk of exposure to mercury not once but multiple times. Arguably, these are very small amounts of mercury but very small amounts of mercury become very dangerous when there is lead involved and the two toxins potentiate. You will recall that at around two years of age, the protective blood-brain barrier forms and a child's brain begins to receive the protection that the adult brain has. It is ironic that the childhood vaccination schedule has children receiving as many as twenty-three vaccine doses, some or all of them potentially containing mercury, prior to acquiring that blood-brain barrier. Many parents report that their toddler was developing typically then regressed into a state of autistic withdrawal and self-injurious behavior immediately and dramatically following their scheduled eighteen-month vaccine.

Is it possible that the dose of mercury contained within the vaccine is the straw that breaks the camel's back, surpassing the threshold of tolerance for a subset of children who have significant amounts of lead already in their system and limited defense against the potentiated toxic effect of *more* mercury?

In the summer of 2001, the US Institute of Medicine delivered its conclusion on the possible link between autism and the mercury preservative that was, and still is, common in many vaccines. The conclusion of the IOM committee was that despite insufficient evidence to prove or disprove a connection, the theory was "biologically plausible," and their recommendation to remove it was put forth.

> The committee also concludes that the evidence is inadequate to accept or reject a causal relationship between thimerosal exposures from childhood vaccines and the neurodevelopmental disorders of autism, ADHD, and speech or language delay. The committee concludes that although the hypothesis that exposure to thimerosal-containing vaccines could be associated with neurodevelopmental disorders is not established and rests on indirect and incomplete information, primarily from analogies with methylmercury and levels of maximum mercury exposure from vaccines given in children, the hypothesis is biologically plausible.[80]

Based on claims by pharmaceutical companies that their products contained only trace amounts of mercury preservative or that their vaccines were mercury free, there was a common assumption that mercury preservative was being phased out or reduced in all vaccines and pharmaceutical products.

That assumption was wrong. Rather, legislation was enacted that protected pharmaceutical companies and vaccine manufacturers from being sued. The legislation did not prohibit the use of mercury in vaccines, and numerous vaccines legally contain it today.

The issue is complicated further. As recently as 2005, random lab tests on vials of "mercury free" vaccines were tested for mercury. According to HAPI, Health Advocacy in the Public Interest, the vials contained both mercury and the potentiating agent, aluminum. The explanation by producing drug companies is that they now only use mercury in the process for creating the vaccines, not as a preservative in the vaccines themselves. Nevertheless, the final vaccines are showing evidence of containing mercury even after it is supposedly filtered out.

An additional problem exists. Multi-vaccine vials that contain mercury preservative put recipients at risk of receiving inconsistent doses. Because the mercury tends to sink to the bottom of the vial, it is not possible to establish which child or individual receiving a vaccine gets more or less of the mercury. Logically, this accounts for some of the differences in vaccine reactions.

Mercury from Dental Amalgam

Vaccines are not the only source of mercury considered to be delivering a massive insult to human biology. The "silver" fillings that dentists have been freely putting in people's mouths are by far the biggest and most dangerous source of mercury when all relative mercury sources are compared.

The controversy over whether or not the forty-nine percent mercury in dental amalgam is safe is not just a modern-day issue. The practice of filling problem teeth with mercury amalgam is not only centuries old, vocal opposition began at least as early as 1840. Concern from within the dental profession itself grew out of the scientific evidence that was gathered from the medicinal use of mercury that had already spanned the three hundred years prior.

The history of ancient Rome detailed how slaves were condemned to slow death in the mercury mines. The fatigue, stomach pain, mental disturbances and tremors were well understood as signs of full-blown adult mercury poisoning. Mercury toxicity in lower exposure levels such as dental amalgam, for example, creates symptoms that are primarily mental, and less obvious to observe and quantify. Hence, claims are ongoing by dentists that mercury amalgam is perfectly safe in a modern-day world that has copious evidence that it is not.

"Mercury got its start in the dental industry in 1826, when a Paris dentist combined it with silver, copper and other metals to create a paste. Seven years later, two brothers in New York City with no dental training began to promote mercury as a cheap alternative to gold fillings."[81] Gold fillings, even today, are challenging and considered a test of a dentist's skill. By comparison, cheap, long-lasting mercury amalgam is quicker and easier to use as filling material.

In his opening address to the inaugural class of the Baltimore College of Dental Surgery in 1840, Dr. Chapin Harris shared this perspective on mercury amalgam: "It is one of the most objectionable articles for filling teeth that can be employed, and yet from the wonderful virtues ascribed to this pernicious compound by those who used it, thousands were induced to try its efficacy."[82] In 1845, the American Society of Dental Surgeons made it mandatory for all members to sign a pledge promising not to use amalgam fillings. As a result of its stance against dental amalgam and the loss of membership that resulted, it was forced to disband. In 1859, the American Dental Association was founded to defend the dental profession from the attack they found themselves under for their use of mercury.[83]

By 1883, the dangers of mercury vapor from dental amalgam were fully in the public eye thanks to the research and writings of E. S. Talbot, entitled *Injurious Effects of Mercury as Used in Dentistry*.[84] Despite what was scientifically revealed as early as 1882 by Talbot and confirmed again in 1926 by German inorganic chemist, Dr. Alfred Stock, the use of mercury amalgam by dentists has expanded with every passing decade.

Amalgam was fast to become the dental standard with the American Dental Association adopting a position of unqualified endorsement of mercury amalgam as safe—the position that it maintains to the present day. In the American Dentists Association's 1972 *Guide to Dental Materials and Devices*, the reader is informed that amalgam does release small amounts of mercury, but that "this evaporation stops as soon as the filling is coated by saliva."[85]

In 1990, the *Journal of the American Dental Association* defended their position on the safety of mercury in dental amalgam, stating that "the strongest and most convincing support we have for the safety of dental amalgam is the fact that each year more than 100 million amalgam fillings are placed in the United States. And since amalgam has been used for more than 150 years, literally billions of amalgam fillings have been successfully used to restore decayed teeth."[86]

The American Dental Association instructed dentists to tell patients who expressed concern about the mercury in amalgam fillings that "the mercury forms a biologically inactive substance when it combines with the other materials."[87] However, researchers from the International Academy of Oral Medicine and Toxicology were able to record their findings in a video clearly documenting mercury vapor being emitted from an amalgam filling.

Likewise, Environment Canada's website, although it does not use the diagnostic term autism, describes the damage that mercury does to adults as well as the unborn child:

> Today, the main effects of mercury exposure to humans are understood to be neurological, renal (kidney), cardiovascular and immunological impacts. Chronic exposure to mercury can cause damage to the brain, spinal cord, kidneys, liver, and developing fetus. Exposure to mercury while in the womb can lead to neurodevelopmental problems in children. Mercury can impair the ability to feel, see, move, and taste, and can cause numbness and tunnel vision. Long-term exposure can lead to progressively worse symptoms and ultimately personality changes, stupor, and in extreme cases, coma or death. Recent findings have described adverse cardiovascular and immune system effects at very low levels.[88]

Despite how safe dentists maintain amalgam is, in 2001 a council of Canadian Ministers of the Environment from each of the provinces and territories coordinated a set of actions for a countrywide standard for dental amalgam waste. (Apparently the same mercury that is safe in our mouths is not safe to be released into the sewer or garbage.)

In Canada, a nation-wide goal was set to achieve a ninety-five percent reduction in mercury releases from dental amalgam waste discharges to the environment. No such reduction of mercury applied to teeth has occurred or been pursued. Only very recently has dental practice evolved to suggest that best practice is not placing fillings in the teeth of small children or women who are pregnant or breastfeeding.

While the Canadian Dental Association maintains its position that mercury amalgam is safe and dentists on both sides of the Canada-US border continue to advocate for its use, the federal government of Canada explains this about the dangers of mercury on its Environment Canada website:

> Prenatal exposure to organic mercury, even at levels that do not appear to affect the mother, may depress the development of the central nervous system and may cause psychomotor retardation for affected children. Mild neurological and developmental delays may occur in infants ingesting methylmercury in breast milk. Affected children may exhibit reduced coordination and growth, lower intelligence, poor hearing and verbal development, cerebral palsy and behavioral problems.[89]

The difficulty reconciling these two positions is more than obvious. Doctor Hal A. Huggins, a leading pioneer in declaring amalgam toxic, proposes that "the financial liability they [dentists] face is far greater than the tobacco suits, and the humiliation they face for knowingly covering up the most effective loss of human potential ever created on the planet is devastating."[90] It may be, therefore, still a while before dentists change their tune and embrace responsibility for the contribution they may have made to autism and a list of other related neurotoxic conditions, Alzheimer's disease and multiple sclerosis to name just two.

We know that the mercury-containing amalgam occupies millions of mouths, young and old, and that dangerous vapor is emitted as a result of chewing, brushing or grinding the teeth together. While there are no studies that we know of at this time, one cannot help wonder what degree of toxic exposure an infant endures with each kiss or word spoken into its face. It seems more likely that we have sealed their fate as autism statistics in the womb before they have ever seen the light of day, and yet it is difficult to entirely discount the possibility that a mouth full of vaporizing mercury, breathed repeatedly in the face of a newborn that already has high levels of lead or other neurotoxins, may have a detrimental impact.

Mercury Exposure Symptoms

The scientific community is not in agreement that mercury, with or without lead or other neurotoxins, is a causal factor in autism. But consider this list of symptoms:

Psychiatric Disturbances: social withdrawal; repetitive behaviors; anxiety; irritability; poor eye contact

Speech/Language Deficits: loss of speech or delayed speech; speech comprehension deficits

Sensory Abnormalities: oral, touch, light and sound sensitivities

Motor Disorders: flapping motions; poor coordination; abnormal gait

Cognitive Impairments: low intelligence; poor memory; difficulty with abstract ideas

Unusual Behaviors: self-injurious; sleep difficulties; ADHD

Physical Disturbances: gastrointestinal disorders; gut dysbiosis; yeast/bacterial overgrowth

Biochemistry: reduced glutathione; decreased detoxification ability of liver; disrupted purine metabolism

Immune System: weakened immune system with increased likelihood of auto-immune response, allergies, and asthma

Central Nervous System Structure: mercury accumulates in amygdala, hippocampus, basal ganglia, and cerebral cortex, which are damaged in autism; mercury also damages Purkinje and granule cells (seen in autism); disruption of neuronal organization

Neurochemistry: decreased serotonin synthesis; elevated norepinephrine and epinephrine; demyelination

Neurophysiology: abnormal EEGs; abnormal vestibular nystagmus response

Gender bias: higher sensitivity/occurrence in males versus females[91]

Is this a list of symptoms of autism or mercury poisoning? The answer is: both. The symptoms for autism and mercury poisoning are virtually the same. To further confound the situation, lead poisoning is often confused for autism as the symptoms also mimic each other.[92]

The factor of potentiation makes it at least plausible that mercury, when combined with lead, causes autism; that autism is the brain's response to being hit not with a single toxic metal, but with the additional cumulative insult of a second and possibly others in a window of vulnerability and susceptibility that is not repeated in the human life cycle. This would logically explain why some mothers with dental amalgam produce children without autism. Or why some children receive vaccines, but not all vaccinated children become autistic.

The world stage, with particular interest paid to China and India, adds another dimension to the in utero or early childhood exposure to neurotoxins. Not so many years ago, autism was virtually unknown in these countries. Since 1999, when the United States made vaccines containing mercury available to them, autism rates have soared. Today, China has more than 1.8 million cases of autism.[93] India, Argentina, Nicaragua and other developing countries that have received vaccines preserved with mercury have experienced exponential increases in rates of autism.

There is one anomalous population within the United States that remains virtually autism-free. Based on the current reported ratios on the incidence of autism (one in 166) in the regular population, this community with but a handful of individuals with autism should statistically have more than one hundred.[94] Is it purely a coincidence that the Amish, a group that does not vaccinate their children and births their babies at home, have beaten the statistical odds on autism?

Whether the lethal dose of mercury is the result of dental amalgam, a vaccine, eye-drops, canned tuna, a broken thermometer or the more probable combination of all of them and more, the solution is obvious. While parents of children who have autism are locked into a sometimes unforgiving reality, those who will produce the next generation may be able to take steps to reduce the chance that their child will have autism or some type of neurotoxic effect.

NOTES

CHAPTER 8

LEAD AND FERTILITY: MEN AND WOMEN

For most couples, fertility is not a problem. For some others, the longing to become a parent remains unfulfilled. Reproductive problems have become common in modern society and some seem to be growing in their incidence. In the United States, infertility is currently estimated to affect more than two million couples. That translates into one couple in twelve finding itself unable to have children. Among other factors, infertility can be caused by problems with ovulation, problems with sperm, age, reproductive infections, damage to reproductive organs, genetic makeup, smoking, drinking, drugs, immunological, anatomic or thyroid problems as well as exposure to radiation and certain chemicals, such as pesticides.

Lead is detrimental to fertility. This was known long ago. Roman women who ingested lead from their food, cosmetics and kitchenware, and who used lead preparations as a contraceptive, suffered from infertility. It has been hypothesized that lead-caused infertility contributed to the fall of the Roman Empire. Luxurious foods such as mulled wine, grape syrup and preserved fruit could only be afforded by the aristocracy. As now, the subtle low-level lead exposure was hard to detect or diagnose and was often confused with other conditions such as alcoholism. As a result, sterility and high rates of miscarriage followed, and the lead-poisoned aristocracy was replaced by their slaves, who did not have access to these culinary luxuries.[95]

In the late 1800s, lead's ability to cause abortion was recognized by women employed in pottery and white lead factories. In 1860, French scientists found that wives of lead workers were more likely to have troubles conceiving and had higher rates of miscarrying. Later, in 1881, lead was reported to cause birth defects as was evidenced by growing numbers of children born with excessively large heads (macrocephaly).[96]

Prenatal exposure to lead starts long before conception. Lead enters the body of parents-to-be in many ways and accumulates over their lifetime. Smaller particles can be breathed in as dust while larger ones, the ones that are too big to get into the lungs, can be coughed up and swallowed. As shown in previous chapters, lead can also be ingested while consuming lead-adulterated food and liquids. As soon as lead gets into the body, it enters the blood system and travels through the soft tissues and organs such as the brain, heart, liver, muscles, kidneys and spleen. After several weeks, more than ninety percent of it moves into the bones and teeth where it remains stored for decades causing disruption in the body's functioning. Thus, past exposures to lead can interfere with a person's ability to have healthy children or to have children at all. Lead exposure, despite its prevalence and known impact, is often overlooked as a factor in the infertility of both men and women.

Male Fertility

Lead accumulates in the male reproductive organs. Its detrimental effects on the male reproductive system have been linked to miscarriages and birth defects that their partners experience, as well as the man's decreased ability to father children.

Lead interferes with male fertility at several sites and levels. It can affect a man's sex drive, ejaculate volume, sperm count and be a reason behind lower percentages of motile sperm or sperm quality. In fact, lead affects all aspects of sperm. Some examples include: sperm's morphology, swimming velocity, total mobility, motility, viability, membrane function, linearity and nuclear DNA integrity.

Lead exposure reduces the sperm count and is the cause of abnormal sperm production. The higher the lead levels in the man's semen, the lower the fertilization rate. For an egg to become fertilized, sperm must first successfully bind to the egg. High lead levels interfere with both the ability of the sperm to bind to the egg and to fertilize the egg. Sperm from men with elevated lead levels is able neither to bind to the egg nor to initiate the reaction that is necessary for it to penetrate the egg's coating. When lead levels are elevated, fewer receptors on the head of the sperm are able to recognize and bind to sugar on the egg.

High lead levels also impede the ability of sperm to penetrate the egg in a process called the acrosome reaction. In such cases, self destructive, "spontaneous" acrosome activity occurs before the sperm reaches the egg.[97] Contrary to what was previously believed, current research shows that not only grown men who are employed in the lead trades have their fertility affected. Men's fertility can be jeopardized without their showing lead toxicity; even low-level lead exposure from household contaminants can damage sperm. Young boys who are exposed to lead during childhood will exhibit impaired sperm production in puberty.[98]

Female Fertility

In women, exposure to environmental toxins can be the cause of a myriad of adverse effects on the reproductive system. They range from impaired evolution of pregnancy to various disabilities of the fetus. Even very low lead levels may cause miscarriage, pre-term delivery, stillbirths and decreased fertility.

Young girls who were exposed to lead in their childhood store most of it in their bones. Later in life, this lead can re-enter the blood and organs under circumstances such as pregnancy and periods of breastfeeding. During these times, the body's calcium levels drop and bones recycle lead back into the bloodstream, redistributing it to the soft tissue organs such as the liver and brain. Since lead can cross the placenta directly to the baby, the fetus can be damaged by the lead deposits contained in the mother's bones and teeth. Thus, a lead exposure in one's childhood can later become adverse results during pregnancy later in life.

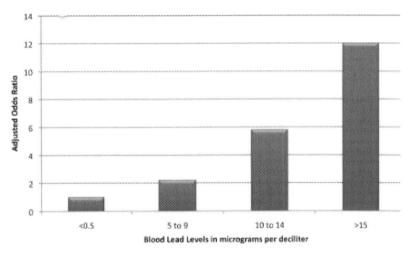

The risk of spontaneous abortion in pregnancy increases with lead exposure

As the lead passes through the placenta into the baby's developing organs and bones, a pregnant woman's exposure to lead puts her unborn baby at many risks. Various malformations are associated with increased maternal levels of lead during pregnancy. They include skin tags and papillae, water accumulation around body cavities, especially in the sac around the testes, benign tumors or birthmarks, lymph tumors, and undescended testicles in males.

Elevated maternal lead levels can also be a cause of decreased birth weight and shortened gestation. It is estimated that each ten micrograms per deciliter of maternal blood lead level translates into a half-week reduction of gestation. It has also been demonstrated that low-level lead exposure may cause a 114-gram decrease in birth weight for every ten micrograms per deciliter increase in maternal blood lead level. When umbilical cord lead levels are compared, children with elevated levels of lead have decreased gestational age compared to those whose blood lead levels are normal.[99] Thus, babies born to mothers with increased bone and blood levels tend to be smaller and gain less weight in the first month of life.

Furthermore, children born to mothers with elevated lead levels experience a whole spectrum of neurological difficulties. When compared to children with normal umbilical cord lead levels, children with elevated levels of lead are behind in mental development. Infants born to mothers with even slightly elevated lead blood levels show abnormal neurological soft signs such as atypical reflexes or sensory responses and decreased muscle tone at birth. Later, they score statistically lower on mental development tests.

Women who are at risk for having increased lead levels during pregnancy should have their blood levels monitored. If their levels are elevated, every attempt should be made to reduce their exposure. There is currently no universal treatment recommended for women with elevated lead levels. Unfortunately, due to their potential for disturbing the growth or development of a fetus or embryo, chelating agents, although effective at reducing lead levels, should not be used during pregnancy.

Nutrition during pregnancy plays an especially important role. Compared to women who do not take prenatal vitamins, women who take vitamins during pregnancy tend to have lower blood-lead levels. Specifically, an inverse association between lead levels and antioxidants such as vitamin E and ascorbic acid was observed.[100] Also, deficiencies in calcium, iron and zinc have been linked to increased lead absorption.

NOTES

CHAPTER 9

OTHER TOXINS:
PARTNERS IN HARM

"Everything is bad for you anyway."

The person who adopts this approach to life is not entirely unjustified. There *are* bad things that affect our health. And there are bad things that are simply unavoidable. The key difference between taking charge of our own lives and the wellbeing of our families is in what we do about the misfortunes that *can* be prevented. Those who resign themselves to a fatalistic approach and choose to live by the mantra, *We are doomed anyway, so why bother?* should beware. They are perpetuating the cycle of precisely the type of damage we are trying to help avoid.

Lead and mercury are not the only players in the growing drama of increasing numbers of children who struggle to learn and behave. There are other antagonists. Currently, over 80,000 different chemicals are used daily on the North American continent. The majority have never been tested for safety, let alone proven safe. Millions and millions of tons of toxins are spat out on the planet daily.

Let's look at the facts. Statistics on world health estimate that, around the world, two billion people have cancer, which kills one in four. Seventeen million people have asthma; four million have Parkinson's disease; 2.5 million have multiple sclerosis; four million have lupus; 4.6 million people have Alzheimer's; forty million have arthritis. In the United States, sixteen percent of the population has been diagnosed with chemical sensitivity. One million Americans have Chronic Fatigue Immune Deficiency Syndrome; twenty-four percent have experienced a mental illness in their lifetime. Thyroid problems are responsible for the highest number of prescribed pharmaceuticals. One in eleven Americans has an overactive bladder and one in six children suffers from a developmental, learning or behavioral disability such as ADHD, mental retardation, autism or birth defects.

Promisingly, there is a growing recognition of the fact that environmental toxins not only exist, but also that they are the root of a multitude of health problems. As more and more studies are generated to show that toxins cause harm, pressure on the companies who produce them mounts. An understanding of the link between toxins, illness and brain damage is becoming mainstream.

What has been presented as a key concept in toxic exposure throughout this book is becoming widely accepted—children in developmental stages are more vulnerable to toxins for a number of reasons. First, the pound for pound exposure to chemicals is greater in small children. Second, the blood-brain barrier is still an immature structure and it allows harmful toxins to permeate the brain. Third, the mechanisms that detoxify and excrete chemicals are not yet fully complete. Additionally, rapidly developing bodies have lower levels of chemical-binding proteins, which makes their organs an easier target for toxins.[101] In its report, *Body Burden—The Pollution in Newborns,* The Environmental Working Group succinctly describes the harm caused by toxins to the unborn child.

> In the month leading up to a baby's birth, the umbilical cord pulses with the equivalent of at least 300 quarts of blood each day, pumped back and forth from the nutrient- and oxygen-rich placenta to the rapidly growing child cradled in a sac of amniotic

fluid. This cord is a lifeline between mother and baby, bearing nutrients that sustain life and propel growth. Not long ago scientists thought that the placenta shielded cord blood—and the developing baby—from most chemicals and pollutants in the environment. But now we know that at this critical time when organs, vessels, membranes and systems are knit together from single cells to finished form in a span of weeks, the umbilical cord carries not only the building blocks of life, but also a steady stream of industrial chemicals, pollutants and pesticides that cross the placenta as readily as residues from cigarettes and alcohol. This is the human "body burden"—the pollution in people that permeates everyone in the world, including babies in the womb.[102]

Damage from toxins is by no means confined to the unborn, but appreciation of the amplified vulnerability of babies in the womb and children is especially critical.

As can be expected, change does not happen overnight. Needleman and Landrigan point out "Each man-made chemical has an industry behind it and it bears a price and a profit."[103] The example of smoking typifies the situation at hand. Even today, when there is ample and irrefutable data to prove that smoking causes harm, the tobacco industry still argues that there is not enough evidence to prove that smoking has detrimental effects on health. And people smoke on.

But change requires something other than an organization or a government body changing its practice and policy. Instead of waiting for a person or organization to take charge, change demands that each of us becomes empowered to make choices and act in ways that will have impact on us and on our families. When faced with the dilemma of environmental toxins and pollutants, we need to become informed, start asking questions and take care of ourselves.

In this book, lead is our focus because the extreme prevalence of it in our lives is matched by a frightening complacency and previous refusal to connect it with the generation of compromised learners who attend our schools and fill our courtrooms. Fortunately, the extensive research on lead and its impact is in the bank. But the trend in research to focus on the damage or impact created by a single toxin undermines our ability to gain a full appreciation of the damage caused by what has become a smorgasbord, a cocktail of toxins that makes accurate portrayal of the impact of any one agent challengeable. As we know from the possible role of lead as a potentiating agent with mercury and other toxins in the epidemic of autism, the synergistic relationships between multiple agents may be exponentially more damaging, yet difficult to pinpoint and prove. This chapter provides an overview of other environmental toxins that are known to have damaging effects on both children and adults.

Heavy Metals

Heavy metals are substances that are toxic even at low concentrations. People are exposed to these metals by drinking polluted water, eating contaminated food and inhaling toxin-filled air. These metals either compete with or mimic other substances, disrupting metabolic function and weakening the body systems. Exposure to these metals can cause serious adverse consequences beyond nervous system damage, including various organ damage, reduced growth and development, and in extreme cases, death.

Researchers ascribe the recent growth in numbers of individuals suffering from a list of autoimmune diseases to heavy metal toxicity. The explanation for these anomalous conditions is that the human system becomes confused and attacks its own cells. This eventually leads to diseases such as rheumatoid arthritis, diabetes, multiple sclerosis, Crohn's disease, lupus, celiac and Grave's disease—the list is long.

People seem content with the explanation that their own body attacks itself. But why would the system attack itself when it is not designed this way? There must be a reason. Something must be interfering with the natural balance. And that is where heavy metals come in. They accumulate in bones, hair, liver and throughout the body. The immune system, on guard like a large, personal army, waits for intruders it does not recognize.

Whereas fever is the immune system's weapon against infection caused by bacteria and viruses, metals are met with antibodies that, when chronic deployment occurs, eventually cause inflammation. Inflammation underlies the symptoms that ultimately manifest themselves as autoimmune diseases in which the body, now confused and stressed, begins attacking itself. The most common and harmful heavy metals include lead, mercury, arsenic, cadmium and manganese. Given the vulnerability of a nervous system and the cumulative nature of toxic load, "safe" levels for these toxins simply do not exist.

Arsenic is a grey metal that occurs naturally in the environment. It is similar to lead in three key aspects. First, once it enters the environment it cannot be destroyed or eliminated. Second, it can harm pregnant women and cross the placenta. Third, chronic exposure to arsenic interferes with child development and assists lead in lowering intelligence.

Exposure to arsenic is mainly from food, but in some areas it is also from drinking water. Arsenic is a byproduct of the burning of arsenate-treated building materials and is also produced during coal combustion. Arsenic is used in various insect sprays, pesticides and cigarettes. It can also be found in soil and in seafood from coastal waters, especially mussels, oysters and shrimp. The effects of arsenic include:

> abdominal pain, anorexia, brittle nails, diarrhea, nausea, vomiting, chronic anemia, burning in the mouth, esophagus, stomach, and bowel, confusion, convulsions, dermatitis, drowsiness, enzyme inhibition, garlicky odor to breath and stool, hair loss, headaches, hyper-pigmentation of nails and skin, increased risk of liver, lung and skin cancers, low grade fever, mucous in the nose and throat, muscle aches and spasms, weakness, nervousness, respiratory tract infection, swallowing difficulty, sweet metallic taste, and throat constriction.[104]

Cadmium is a soft, bluish metal that is used in the production of re-chargeable batteries, metal plating and paint pigments, and as a stabilizer in the manufacture of plastic and other synthetics. Cadmium ends up in the atmosphere following several pathways. It is released into the atmosphere by mining, fossil fuel burning, manufacturing operations, as well as medical and municipal waste incinerators. It is contained in sewage sludge and phosphate fertilizers.

After cigarettes, food is the most common source of cadmium. An average adult consumes ten to thirty micrograms of cadmium daily. Leafy vegetables and grain crops readily absorb cadmium contained in the soil, the residue of cadmium-enriched fertilizers. It accumulates in shellfish from coastal waters. Other food sources include candy, drinking water, evaporated milk, instant coffee, processed meat, refined grains, flour and cereals. Cadmium is also contained in dental alloys, cigarette smoke, marijuana and silver polish.

Research on effects of cadmium has shown that the metal has detrimental effects on a developing nervous system. It can be toxic to the growing brain either directly or indirectly.

> During pregnancy cadmium may interfere with placental and essential enzyme function or the availability of essential trace elements or other nutrients. Neonatal exposures alter neurotransmitter levels, including norepinephrine, dopamine, serotonin, and acetylcholine. Cadmium exposure is also associated with increased free radical production in tissues resulting in cell membrane damage and changes in a variety of other physiological functions.[105]

One study found a correlation between hyperactivity and elevated levels of lead and cadmium in hair. Another study conducted among 149 children aged five to sixteen, evidenced a correlation between elevated lead and cadmium levels and reduced verbal and performance IQ levels. Yet more research, showed that lead and cadmium affected different aspects of intelligence. While lead levels were more strongly correlated with reduced performance IQ, elevated cadmium levels caused reduced verbal IQ.[106] Elevated cadmium levels have also been shown to interfere with children's perceptual and motor development.[107]

Other effects of cadmium include alcoholism, alopecia, anemia, arthritis (osteo and rheumatoid), bone disease, bone pain, cancer, cardiovascular disease, cavities, cerebral hemorrhage, cirrhosis, diabetes, digestive disturbances, emphysema, enlarged heart, flu-like symptoms, growth impairment, headaches, high cholesterol, hyperkinetic behavior, hypertension, hypoglycemia, impotence, inflammation, infertility, kidney disease, learning disorders, liver damage, lung disease, migraines, nerve cell damage, osteoporosis, prostate dysfunction, reproductive disorders, schizophrenia, and stroke.[108]

Manganese is a grey metal that is found naturally in the earth's crust. Unlike lead or mercury, some manganese is essential for the human body to function properly. Manganese works as a catalyst in several essential enzymatic processes; it is a necessary trace nutrient required in all live organisms.

In industry, it is used as a pigment and as an oxidation chemical. Manganese replaced lead in unleaded gasoline as the octane booster and anti-knocking agent. Consequently, manganese is now everywhere.

The manganese used in gasoline releases manganese compounds into the atmosphere. As expected, these discharged particles end up being inhaled. According to a study from 1996, manganese particles bypass the body's general circulation and end up directly in the brain.[109]

Except for occupational-related exposure, the most common source of manganese is food. Unfortunately, following the logic that human breast milk is deficient in manganese, it is added regularly to infant formulas. Soy-derived formulas already contain high levels of naturally-occurring manganese. However, since studies show that compared to adults children absorb much more and excrete much less manganese, and since it has been shown to travel freely through the blood brain barrier to accumulate in the developing brain, the logic behind supplementation of baby food with manganese seems obscure.[110]

The most critical health effect of manganese is that, even at very low levels, it causes brain damage. As with lead, exposure to this metal during the period of brain development results in neurological damage that manifests as hyperactivity and learning disabilities. The link between hyperactivity or learning disabilities and elevated levels of manganese in hair has been documented by several studies. The research shows clearly that the level of manganese in hair correlates with higher incidence of learning disabilities and hyperactivity with and without attention deficit.[111]

The symptoms of manganese poisoning include tremor and movement disorders that can be followed by "manganese madness," a condition manifesting itself in compulsive singing, fighting and running. Although there are some differences, the movement disorder characteristic of manganism is similar to that of Parkinson's disease.[112]

Mercury is a toxic heavy metal. Once in the environment, elemental mercury is transformed into organic forms that accumulate in the human body, animals, fish and plants. Millions of pounds of mercury are released in the atmosphere yearly, primarily by coal-powered plants, waste incineration, as well as various mining and smelting activities.

Mercury is a cause of many adverse health effects. Most notably, it harms pregnant women, their unborn babies, and young children. Substantial fetal exposure to mercury causes serious mental disabilities affecting gait and sensory processing. Even amounts considered safe by the World Health Organization cause permanent damage to the embryonic nervous system of fetuses that later results in brain dysfunction related to language processing, memory and attention span (see chapter 7).

Other Toxins

Bisphenol A is a synthetic chemical compound that is an ingredient of many polymers and polymer additives. It is used in the production of polycarbonate plastic and epoxy resins, two versatile materials that are used in the manufacturing of many products. According to an estimate for 2002 by the US Chemical Market Associates, the global production of bisphenol A reached 2.8 million tons.

Bisphenol A is used in the production of reusable food and drink containers such as plastic water bottles and baby bottles. It is also contained in food and beverage can linings, electrical and electronic equipment, digital media such as CDs and DVDs, automobiles, sports and safety equipment, paints, adhesives, dental sealants and composites, and a multitude of other products.[113]

Bisphenol A has been found to mimic estrogen and thus interfere with functioning of hormones. Bisphenol A that comes in contact with food is of particular concern. Mounting animal studies suggest that the chemical is detrimental to human health. One study has found that exposure to bisphenol A may increase the risk of developing breast cancer. It has also been indicated as playing a role in increasing the risk of cancer following an in utero exposure. It may also impede fertility and contribute to children's behavioral problems. A study by the US Centers for Disease Control and Prevention found bisphenol A in ninety-five percent of the tested population.[114]

Dioxin is a general term that describes hundreds of chemicals that are amongst the most noxious known to science. Dioxin is highly persistent in the environment and poses a very serious threat to human health. It is a by-product of many industrial processes such as waste incineration, manufacturing of pesticides and other chemicals, secondary copper smelting, as well as chlorine-based pulp and paper bleaching.[115] Dioxin was the primary toxic component of Agent Orange, a plant-killer used in the war in Vietnam.

As with cadmium and manganese, exposure to dioxins is mainly through the food we consume. Dioxin accumulates in animal fat, with the highest levels in animals that live the longest. The amount of dioxin also depends on where the animal is in the food chain; the higher the position in the food chain, the higher the dioxin concentration. Ninety percent of the dioxin intake in a typical North American diet comes from meat and dairy products.[116] Because of its fat content, breast milk typically contains high levels of dioxin, leaving breast-fed infants with correspondingly high dioxin intake.

Dioxin has made headlines in several countries. In the spring of 1978, the residents of Love Canal, a small town in Niagara Falls, New York discovered that over twenty thousand tons of chemical waste from a dumpsite was leaking into their community. The dumpsite was once a canal built by William T. Love to connect the upper and lower Niagara River. Before completing his ambitious project, Mr. Love ran out of money and the forsaken canal was sold and used as a municipal and chemical dumpsite.

From 1920 to 1953, over two hundred different chemicals were deposited there. They included toxic substances such as dioxin, PCBs, solvents and heavy metals. After the site was filled, it was covered and sold to the Niagara Falls Board of Education. An elementary school and approximately 800 single-family homes and 240 apartments were built next to the dump.[117] What was intended to be a dream community was ultimately abandoned, a ghost town, but only after illness on a tragic scale: miscarriages, leukemia, cancer and birth defects became the community's norm.

In the 1980s, the town of Times Beach, Missouri was evacuated due to dioxin contamination. This time the toxin came from waste oil used to spray roads to control dust. This technique of controlling dust was first used in horse stables and caused the death of sixty-two horses in 1971. When more horses died in following years, stable owners contacted the US Environmental Protection Agency seeking help. It turned out that the soil in the vicinity of Times Beach contained dangerously high levels of dioxin. Eventually, a dioxin task force was established by President Ronald Reagan, and in 1985 the entire town of Times Beach was evacuated and abandoned.

Dioxin adversely affects brain development. Delays in the area of psychomotor development, attention deficits, changes in behavior, as well as impaired cognitive development such as decreased IQ have been documented in a number of animal and human studies. Significant, direct dioxin exposure has resulted in Chloracne, a severe skin disease with acne-like lesions that occur mainly on the face and upper body. Other effects of exposure to dioxin include skin rashes, skin discoloration, excessive body hair and liver damage.[118]

A major concern of direct exposure is the link between dioxin and cancer. Additionally, animal studies suggest that prolonged exposure even to low levels of dioxin may compromise reproduction.

Toxic Flame Retardants, polybrominated diphenyl ethers, or PBDEs are materials that resist fire. They are commonly used in household items such as carpets, mattresses, sofas, television sets, computers, electronics and motor vehicles. In recent years, they have been detected in our bodies; they have been found in breast milk and blood, including umbilical cord blood.

PBDEs have been indicated as damaging to the neurological, reproductive, immune, and hormonal systems, causing conditions such as learning and memory difficulties, cancers, heart, lung and kidney problems, skin irritations, and sudden infant death syndrome. Some PBDEs have been linked to brain and thyroid problems in laboratory rodents.

PBDEs do not permanently bind with the products they are added to so they continuously migrate and accumulate in the fat tissue of people and animals. According to research, human PBDE levels are doubling every two to five years. Compared to residents of other continents, North Americans carry forty times more PBDEs in their systems.[119]

Polychlorinated Biphenyls, PCBs, are a class of 209 synthetic chemicals that contain atoms of chlorine. Unlike dioxins that were produced unintentionally as the by-product of other processes, PCBs were produced for many years for specific industrial purposes. PCBs were widely used as lubricants and liquid insulators in electric transformers. They were also used in ballasts and fluorescent lights.

Due to their extreme toxicity, production of PCBs has been banned in many countries. However, like many other toxins, once released the PCBs persist in the environment decade after decade; they reside in air, soil and water. They accumulate and move up the food chain: "from the sediments in the bottom of lakes and rivers they are taken up by worms, shellfish, catfish, eels and other bottom-feeding animals. When those animals in turn are eaten by game fish, the PCBs accumulate to even higher levels in the fatty tissues of those predator species. Finally, when eagles, bears, or humans, the predators who are at the top of the food chain, eat fish, they can accumulate high levels of PCBs."[120]

Because PCBs bio-accumulate in fatty tissue, their highest accumulation is in dairy products, fish, beef and pork. Hence, one of the main concerns about the exposure to PCBs by breastfeeding women is that the toxin that is stored over the years in fatty tissue becomes mobilized and transferred through the breast milk to the infant. In some situations, an infant can accumulate an amount of these toxins equivalent to an adult's body burden. Compared to the average adult daily intake of PCBs, breastfed infants receive sixty times that amount.[121]

The US Environmental Protection Agency is well aware that PCBs have significant toxic properties that negatively affect the nervous system. Newborn monkeys exposed to PCBs showed significant and lasting deficits in neurological development that included visual recognition, short term memory and learning in general. Studies conducted on human populations suggest effects similar to those reported in monkeys.[122] Tested years after exposure, children who were exposed to PCBs in utero have IQ deficits, hyperactivity and attention deficits. PCBs were first identified as harmful to the developing fetus in late 1960 in Japan when PCB-contaminated rice oil was consumed by pregnant women.

A similar incident took place in the following decade in Taiwan. Along with having low birth weight, dark-pigmented skin, as well as swollen eyelids and gums, children born to mothers exposed to PCBs developed neurological disabilities. When tested for academic aptitude, exposed children had lower IQ scores. They were also hyperactive and experienced behavior problems.[123]

Two studies investigated the effects of PCBs in children born to mothers who consumed contaminated fish, one from Lake Michigan and the other one from Lake Ontario. Both studies reported that when compared to children with low PCB exposure, children who received the most exposure were several times as likely to achieve low scores on IQ and attention span tests. Some of the common effects of PCBs in children described by theses studies include abnormal reflexes and startle responses, impaired visual recognition, disturbances in neuromotor activity, neurodevelopmental delays, as well as impairments of higher cognitive functions and learning.[124]

Pesticides are used by most people regularly. They can be found virtually everywhere. They are used to stave off insects so that a beautiful sunset can be enjoyed, they are applied to front yards so that their owners can be proud of their weed-free lawns, and they are snapped around the necks of pets so that they are not bothered by fleas. Pesticides are an ingredient in insect repellents and sprays, rat and other rodent poisons, products that kill mould and mildew, treated wood, and pool chemicals. Pesticides are used in most kitchen, laundry and bath disinfectants and sanitizers. Pesticide residue is common on our fruits, vegetables and other foods. The irony of the use of pesticides is that while developed to get rid of organisms considered harmful to the wellbeing of humans, pesticides inadvertently hurt the very individuals whose lives they were developed to improve. In their quest to protect their homes, crops and selves from pests, humans have saturated themselves with thousands of chemicals while knowing very little about the associated health effects.

According to the Canadian Organization of Physicians for the Environment (CAPE), "pesticides are among the most widely used chemicals in the world, and also among the most dangerous to human health. They are a leading cause of poisonings (...) and have been estimated to account for thousands of deaths each year globally."[125]

The US Environmental Protection Agency estimates that every year over five billion pounds of pesticides is used worldwide with over one fifth of this amount being utilized in the United States. The US Centers for Disease Control and Prevention reports that more than ninety percent of Americans carry a mixture of pesticides in their bodies. In a study conducted by the Centers for Disease Control and Prevention, the blood and urine collected from a random sample of Americans contained 148 various chemicals of which forty-three were pesticides.[126] In a similar study by the Environmental Working Group, fetal cord blood of healthy infants was tested. The results obtained revealed that on average, the blood of a single umbilical cord contains 287 different chemicals.[127] One common organophosphate insecticide has been measured in the urine of ninety percent of American children.[128]

Whatever definition of pesticides one decides to use, one thing is certain: pesticides are toxic by design. The evidence of the harmful effects of pesticides is mounting. Animal tests on one class of commonly used pesticides confirm that even a small single dose on a critical day of development can be a cause of hyperactivity and permanent alterations in the brain's neurotransmitter receptor levels. One commonly used pesticide reduces the process of DNA synthesis in the developing brain, causing deficits in cell numbers. Children exposed to a variety of pesticides in various agricultural communities show impaired stamina, poor coordination, memory difficulties, and a diminished capacity to represent familiar subjects in drawings.[129]

Phthalates, also called phthalate esters, are a group of versatile synthetic chemicals used mainly to increase the flexibility of plastics or to prolong the life of fragrances. They have been widely used for the last several decades as an ingredient in many products and it is estimated that over a billion pounds of various phthalates is produced each year.[130] They are used in hundreds of products including lubricants, vinyl flooring, carpets, emulsion paint, adhesives, insect repellents, plastics such as toys, plastic wrap, bottles, food containers, food packaging and rain gear. They are also found in personal care products such as cosmetics, deodorants, perfumes, nail polish, shampoo, hair spray powder, lotion and infant wipes. Until 1999, they were utilized in the production of teethers, pacifiers and soft rattles.

Phthalates are also an ingredient in virtually all foods, including baby formula,[131] potato chips, chocolate bars, meat, fish, eggs, cakes, fats and confectionery products.[132] They are present in various water bodies including drinking water.[133] In these products, phthalates are not chemically attached, and thus are continuously released either through the air or through the process of leaching into liquids. Eventually, they end up being inhaled, ingested or transferred through skin.[134]

Recent research suggests that phthalates can damage lungs, liver and kidneys, as well as interfere with endocrine and reproductive systems. The European Union has so far banned the use of six phthalates that were added to products intended for the use of children.[135] Since in the United States there is no legislation limiting their use, and manufacturers are not required to list phthalates on product ingredient lists, it is impossible to know which merchandise contains phthalates.

Solvents are exactly what the name describes; substances that can dissolve grease and other fatty materials. Solvents can be found in every household. Toluene and turpentine are used as paint thinners. Acetone, methyl acetate and ethyl acetate are found in nail polish removers and glue. Hexane and petrol ether eliminate stains. Tetrachloroethylene is used as an active ingredient in dry-cleaning solutions. Terpenes are ingredients in detergents. Ethanol is added to perfumes and consumed as an alcoholic beverage. Toluene and xylene are contained in gasoline and its vapors. Toluene is also a common ingredient used in glues, inks, paints and various cleaning agents.

Organic solvents are common in a variety of activities and industries. Millions and millions of pounds of solvents are released into the environment annually. Exposure to organic solvents during development can cause a spectrum of disorders that include structural birth defects, hyperactivity, attention deficits, and decreased IQ, as well as learning and memory deficiencies. One of the most common solvents, alcohol, is a proven fetal toxicant that leads to impulsive behavior and permanent deficits in memory and IQ, as well as poor school performance and impaired social skills. Studies show that alcohol exposure to a fetus causes reduced brain weight, impaired maturation, loss of certain cells and damaged synaptic connections.[136]

We have long since reached a point in time when there is no room to argue that any of these toxins are safe. Indeed, even the tobacco and pharmaceutical giants are left only to claim that "there is not enough *evidence*" to say their products are unsafe. That is quite a different matter than suggesting that they *do not cause harm*.

On the one hand we are indignant that our world has been poisoned without our permission or our knowledge. On the other, we are the consumers with the voracious appetite for the gasoline and energy that makes our world so wonderful—for snow-white two-ply and unlimited flushes; for bug-free evenings on maintenance-free sundecks. The question then becomes, what changes can we make? How can we maintain a modern, mainstream lifestyle, but minimize our exposure to the toxins that will ultimately undermine the quality of life we desire? Lead is detectable and we can remove or avoid it without turning our lives upside down. By gaining a better understanding of what kinds of products and places are high risk for lead, we can check them and ensure our safety with surprising ease.

NOTES

CHAPTER 10

BREAKING THE CYCLE: AVOIDING AND MINIMIZING EXPOSURE

Here in North America we have a pretty fair exchange program going with countries on the other side of the globe—China, for example. We sent them vaccines containing mercury and our technological waste contaminated with lead and mercury. They returned the favor by sending us lead-contaminated toys and consumer products and mercury plumes from their energy plants that sail here on the jet stream. This book is not about taking on China and its world-polluting energy needs, especially if we have not turned some lights off and adjusted the thermostat at home. This is a book about becoming empowered as an individual or a family to make small changes that will yield life-altering benefits.

The investment of time, money and effort required to eliminate and reduce daily lead exposure is small. The benefit to each of us, our families and tomorrow's children, is truly great.

For readers who are young and thinking about starting a family, the benefits of eliminating and reducing lead now are clear. Those who have had their children and who are feeling that it is too late for them should reconsider. Heavy metal toxicity plays a significant role in the development of Alzheimer's and many autoimmune diseases. This is serious business at whatever stage of life each of us is at.

We hope that by now the main message of our book has become apparent: *lead damage is preventable*. Nowadays, no one needs to be exposed to lead and to suffer its harmful effects. Our children can be protected from the cycle of damage caused by lead. What you have learned in this book will empower you to take action. This chapter will guide you through some simple steps that can be taken to either reduce or prevent lead exposure.

It is important to remember that there is no insignificant amount of lead exposure. It is the nature of how we live and work that if there is a trace amount exposure in our midst, the likelihood that we will reencounter it tomorrow, the next day, and the next, is great. We are creatures of habit; drinking from the same tap, opening and closing the same window, buying and consuming the same brands. A bottle of baby formula made with water from a tap containing a minimal amount of lead must be seen as the gallons of water and dangerous total of accumulated lead that is actually consumed over months and years. The trace amount of lead ingested after each application of lipstick is by no means insignificant when lipstick, applied daily, becomes pounds of cosmetics over a lifetime. And why not go out of our way to steer clear of one-time accidental exposures? They simply add to our lead load and the consequential damage that will ultimately rob from our quality of life. Every little bit hurts!

It's in What You Eat

Proper nutrition plays an important role in protection from the harmful effects of lead. Since lead mimics calcium, human bodies are tricked into storing lead in the system. Once lead enters the body, some of it becomes eliminated via the bladder and bowels. What remains enters the blood system and is later stored in the bones, organs and brain tissue.

Eating right can reduce the amount of lead that becomes absorbed by the human body. While some fat is necessary for proper health and development, especially for children under the age of two, foods with high fat content encourage lead absorption. Foods that need to be consumed in moderation include fast foods, fatty meats, chips, pastries, bacon and butter.

Experiments conducted with adult volunteers showed that lead absorption is much lower (six percent) right after a person has eaten. Participants who had not eaten for a day absorbed sixty to eighty percent lead. Since lead is absorbed more readily on an empty stomach, it is important to consume regular, healthy meals each day.

Foods rich in iron, vitamin C and calcium decrease the amount of lead that the body will store.

Iron is notoriously low in the North American diet, especially in children one to two years old and in women. There is evidence that iron helps block lead absorption in the gastrointestinal system. Studies of lead poisoned children suggest that iron supplements improve development assessment scores. Substantial amounts of iron are contained in foods such as beans, peas, lentils, spinach, dried peaches, prune juice, wholesome breakfast cereals (whole wheat, wheat flakes, farina, and oats), almonds, liver, clams, lean meats, as well as pumpkin, sunflower and squash seeds.

Calcium has been shown to reduce absorption and retention of lead, as well as lower blood lead levels. In one study, lactating women were supplemented daily with 1200 milligrams of calcium over a period of six months. Calcium supplementation produced blood lead level reduction in all women. The effect was most pronounced in women with the highest bone lead levels; their blood lead level declined by as much as sixteen percent.[137] Some common sources of calcium are dairy products, turnip greens, spinach, sardines, salmon, blackstrap molasses, almonds, peanuts, broccoli and shrimp.

A word of caution: some calcium supplements especially the ones that have dolomite, oyster shells, bone meal and coral calcium listed on their labels may contain lead (see chapter 3).

Vitamin C is also crucial. It not only supports the process of ridding the body of heavy metals, it improves iron absorption as well. Vitamin C has been found to decrease blood lead level concentration. A study published by the *Journal of the American Medical Association* reported that individuals with high levels of vitamin C intake had lower lead levels in their bloodstream. The data showed that children with the higher vitamin C intake were eighty-nine percent less likely to have elevated blood lead levels compared with youths with the lowest intake. When it came to mature populations, the study reported that adults with the highest vitamin C intake were sixty-five to sixty-eight percent less likely to have elevated blood lead levels compared with adults with the lowest intake.[138]

Foods that provide significant amounts of this vitamin are citrus fruits (oranges, lemons, grapefruit), cantaloupe, strawberries, kiwi fruit, tomatoes, broccoli, cabbage, collard greens, and bell peppers.

Guidelines for avoiding lead exposure from consumables and from food containers:

- Avoid canned foods from foreign countries with less strict regulations and inspection standards
- Avoid storing acidic or alcoholic food and beverage in ceramic, crystal or pewter containers, hand-painted china and imported pottery
- Avoid using cracked or rustic pottery which may be improperly fired
- Avoid reusing wrapping such as bread bags
- Avoid wrapping food so that it touches color printing inks
- Avoid storing food in PVC (Polyvinylchloride) containers
- Avoid using imported coffee urns and kettles
- Avoid using hot tap water for cooking
- Avoid drinking water from a garden hose
- Avoid using folk remedies
- Avoid consuming waterfowl and game
- Avoid smoking or staying in areas where others are smoking
- Carefully research ingredients in products for diarrhea, especially before giving to children

- Wet wipe surfaces before preparing food
- Wash hands before preparing and eating food
- Wash all fruit and vegetables before eating or cooking
- Use one percent vinegar solution or other store-bought produce cleaning product to remove lead-containing residue on fruit or vegetables
- Wash leafy vegetables thoroughly; discard outer leaves
- Peel all root vegetables
- Never use warm or hot tap water to prepare baby formula
- Ensure that children do not ingest bath water, especially if the bathtub is worn or chipped
- Beware of imported candy, spices and dried fruit such as raisins
- Minimize chocolate consumption
- When opening a bottle of wine that has a foil wrapping, remove the entire foil, wipe the neck, rim and top of the cork with a wet cloth before uncorking the bottle

Products for Children

There are many products on the market designed specifically for children. Adults in the past assumed they were safe, given children's susceptibility to lead damage and the responsibility of manufacturers. Many products targeted at children are not lead-free.

Guidelines for avoiding lead exposure from toys, accessories and other items intended for children's use:

- Avoid ready-made papier-mâché as it may contain lead from pigments in colored printing inks
- Avoid giving keys to children to play with
- Avoid PVC bibs; ensure children do not put bibs in their mouths or chew on them
- Avoid using baby talcum and baby creams that contain zinc oxide
- Beware of PVC lunchboxes
- Research and buy lead-free alternatives for toys

- Do not give children imported crayons or sidewalk chalk
- Newsprint and wrapping paper are not toys: avoid giving them to children to play with
- Check the recall lists regularly. These are most easily obtained from Internet websites belonging to federal regulatory bodies or government agencies.

Personal Hygiene

Good daily hygiene goes a long way in minimizing and preventing lead exposure that, with accumulation over time, can become significant. While such practice is obvious, many associate good hygiene with protection against germs. It is an important element in avoiding and reducing lead exposure as well.

Guidelines for personal hygiene practices that prevent lead exposure:

- Avoid progressive hair dyes
- Avoid imported cosmetics
- Wash hands with soap regularly
- Wash hands before eating, after playing with pets and working or playing outside
- Shower to remove lead from skin and hair
- Dry hands after washing as dust sticks to wet hands
- Use lead-free personal care products
- Minimize the use of products that contain zinc oxide

Housekeeping

Dusting and vacuuming contribute to lead distribution in the home and need to be done in such manner that the amount of dust released into the air is minimized. Airborne dust can be inhaled or will settle back on surfaces. Wet-wiping and mopping are safer than dusting with a feather duster and sweeping with a broom. Waiting at least an hour after vacuuming before mopping maximizes the amount of dust removed with a wet mop. Wet-wiping of furniture and fittings after vacuuming removes lead from surfaces.

Unlike regular vacuum cleaners that do not filter fine lead particles, vacuum cleaners equipped with High Efficiency Particulate Air (HEPA) filters and ducted vacuum systems help prevent the release of dust particles into the air. Vacuuming less often lessens the amount of lead that is ingested from airborne dust.

A three bucket cleaning system is recommended by the US Environmental Protection Agency where there are concerns about lead:

Prepare three buckets (one for detergent, one for clean water and one for used water), two mops or rags, and a lead-specific cleaning detergent such as liquid sugar soap.

Directions:
1. Place mop into detergent solution and wipe area
2. Squeeze into empty bucket
3. Place second mop into clean water; wipe area and squeeze into empty bucket
4. Replace water every room or every half hour, whichever comes first
5. Pour water down toilet
6. Start at top floor and furthest corner from the door

This method is not required for everyday cleaning but is advised in situations such as after renovations or major cleans.

Carpets and other soft surfaces such as curtains attract dust. They are difficult to keep dust-free. Once contaminated, carpets are impossible to be rid of dust completely. Large amounts of lead can be released while removing old carpet. Spraying the carpet with water helps keep the dust down. In general, hard surfaces collect less dust and the accumulated dust can be readily removed.

Pets can bring large amounts of lead-containing dust inside. They need to be brushed and bathed often. Washing hands after playing with an animal is essential.

Items frequently used by children such as **soft toys and blankets** need to be laundered regularly. Anything that cannot be laundered can be kept clean by wet-wiping frequently.

Occupational and Hobby-Related Lead Exposure

The following recommendations were developed by the US Safety and Health Assessment and Research for Prevention Program for people who are exposed to lead in the workplace. These instructions are also suitable for individuals who are exposed to lead as a result of their hobbies.

- Wash hands and face before eating, drinking or smoking
- Eat, drink and smoke only in areas free of lead dust and fumes
- Insure ventilation is adequate or that a properly fitted respirator is in use when lead is present
- Avoid stirring up lead-containing dust with dry sweeping or blowing; wet cleaning and vacuuming with a closed system or HEPA filter are safer
- Protect home and family; do not shake off dusty clothes inside
- Use separate work clothes and shoes while at work
- Keep street clothes in a clean place; do not wear work clothes or shoes/boots at home
- If possible, shower at work before returning home
- Launder work clothes at work or if at home, wash and dry them separately from non-work clothes. To protect against cross-contamination, rinse out the washing machine after laundering work clothes

Outdoors

Play areas where lead is present can be made exposure-safe. The easiest way is by creating a barrier. This can be done by covering exposed soil patches with mulch such as pebbles, grass and shrubbery. As mulch does not stay in place permanently, these barriers need to be maintained regularly. Mats can be installed under swing sets where grass becomes worn and dirt is exposed. In order to eliminate the possibility of lead exposure completely, the contaminated soil needs to be removed and replaced with a new batch of non-contaminated soil. Sandboxes need to be filled with sand that is specifically lead-free and covered while not in use.

Home gardens may be a source of lead exposure. To minimize the uptake of lead from soil, pH levels of garden soil must remain above 6.5. This can be achieved by adding lime or organic matter such as composted leaves or non-acid peat to the soil. Lead binds with organic matter in the soil and becomes less readily available for produce. As in the case of play areas, soil in home gardens can be removed and replaced with clean, fresh soil.

Renovation, Remodelling and Lead

The riskiest practices while renovating include sanding, scraping or using a heat gun to remove leaded paint. The US Consumer Product Safety Commission advises that there is no safe do-it-yourself method to remove lead-containing paint and that it should be left to expert contractors. In the United States, contractors are obligated by law to provide a lead hazard information pamphlet, *Protect Your Family from Lead in Your Home*, to residents prior to commencing any renovation or remodeling project. Moreover, contractors are required to obtain a declaration from the occupants or property owners if lead-containing paint has ever been identified at the site. The worksite must be set up so that the work zone is contained and dust and debris are confined. If in close proximity to the worksite, windows, doors and vents need to be sealed. Eating, drinking or smoking should be avoided in the work zone. At the end of each day, the worksite must be thoroughly cleaned. Waste should be placed in heavy-duty plastic bags, tightly sealed with duct tape and disposed of following appropriate local or federal regulations. These measures apply to interior and exterior renovation projects.

NOTES

CHAPTER 11

TACKLING THE PROBLEM

Appreciative that your time is valuable, your money is precious, and your energy is limited, we have honed a three-step process that minimizes the drain on each. We recommend that you complete step one before moving to step two, and so on, with the emphasis on thoroughness and follow-through. Our hope for you is a well-executed assessment and a thoughtful, realistic plan. We have designed an easy to follow inventory to guide you through the process from testing to action plan.

STEP ONE: Test your water

The Lead Inventory begins with testing the lead in your water because it will most likely be the biggest source of lead you and your family are ingesting on a daily or regular basis. There are other important lead sources in steps two and three but taking action to protect your family from potential daily sources of lead in water is straightforward and may yield a degree of safeguarding that is simply invaluable. Getting organized and being thorough is the key. The following instructions will walk you through the process.

Deciding what to test

The highest priority sources are those used for drinking water on a frequent or regular basis. Water sources for brushing teeth, hand washing, bathing and showering are also important sources that should be tested. Faucets are significant for lead-contaminated water but they may not be the only sources. How do you make your morning tea or coffee? Is your kettle or coffee maker a lead source? If you have a regular stop for coffee, the water they use may be a problem, just as the coffee urn at work may be.

Cats and dogs will lap up the puddle of water left in the shower or bath and are more than happy to drink out of the toilet bowl. Some porcelain fixtures contain lead, as can the bases of shower stalls or bathtubs. Perhaps there are outdoor sources unique to your property that your pets frequent when they are thirsty.

Once you ascertain that the water supply to your washing machine is free of lead, you might consider testing the water late in the first wash cycle, but prior to the rinse cycle, if you or a member of your family has lead-contaminated work clothes that you routinely throw in with the regular wash load.

Water dispensers have become commonplace in homes and commercial settings. Many offer a ready source of hot water, as well as cold, with water sitting in contact with taps and storage tanks for long periods of time. Although it may seem like stating the obvious to some, boiling water will not reduce or eliminate any lead it might contain.

Target and test anything that holds the water you, your children or your pets drink or wash with regularly as it might be a potential lead source. If the lead-free water from your tap is being poured into a kettle made with solder that leaks lead, then you still have the problem. Heated water simply leaches the lead faster making kettles and coffee makers all the more dangerous if they contain lead. Check them! Similarly, if your refrigerator's water or ice-dispenser bypasses a filter system, then test that too.

Make a list of all of your water sources below. Ask yourself: where do you and your family spend your time? Consider your office, or work site, neighbors' and relatives' houses, daycare, school, restaurant, coffee drive-through, etc.

List them here as you think of them:

_____   _____

_____   _____

_____   _____

_____   _____

_____   _____

_____   _____

_____   _____

Now, with your list drafted, go back and prioritize; number according to the most urgent and important to test. Sources you drink from will be highest priority, with who uses them and how often being factors in how you prioritize. Having a sense of which sources are most critical will assist you in developing your response plan later.

Sampling technique

Obtaining three samples from each faucet may assist in determining whether the lead source is the pipes or the tap. Take a "first draw" sample from the cold-water tap after it has been left unused overnight, or at least six to eight hours. Take a second cold water "flush" sample after running the water for long enough to remove any standing water from the pipes. If there is a hot water tap, obtain a third sample by running it until the water is hot to the touch. Samples should be 250 ml (one cup) in volume.

For testing kettles and coffee makers, make sure you begin with water you have verified as completely free of lead. Test water that has sat overnight in the unit. Also test water that has been heated or boiled once it has cooled down and you can safely handle it. Label the location and type of sample, as well as the date, and note each in the inventory located in appendix 1.

Options for testing

There may be a free local water-testing program in the municipality or county where you live. You may also call your municipal or county water distribution office and request individual testing. Look on your water bill to find their contact information. Alternatively, a provincially or state-certified laboratory is the recommended option for testing lead levels in your water. The cost ranges widely, so call around.

Home kits are available at hardware stores and from the Internet. Be cautious and do your research to ensure that you choose one that is sensitive enough and consistent to provide you with the accuracy you need.

Interpretation of results

Note the results of the testing in the inventory. If the test results of the drinking water from your faucets show lead higher than fifteen parts per billion, then your local health department will wish to know. The only truly "safe" level of lead, however, is a reading of zero. If your results reveal *any* presence of lead, a response plan for that source should be developed.

Developing a response plan

Once you have collected your test results, identify which water sources require the highest priority response, based on the frequency and type of water use and the amount of lead detected. You can respond by choosing to eliminate the lead source completely, or you may decide to simply take steps to reduce your exposure to it. We recommend that you research options and solutions for your unique situation. Your personal financial resources will be a factor in deciding how you wish to proceed. Most importantly, you will need to identify what requires immediate attention, what you plan to do, who will be responsible for it, the timeline for completion, and the cost. Here are some examples of options for eliminating and reducing lead in water:

- Flush pipes to drain water before drinking.
- Use a lead filtering jug; in-home water treatment devices can be certified through the US Water Quality Association in the United States or the Canadian Water Quality Association in Canada.
- Install an under-sink filter system. Since not all water filtration systems remove dissolved lead, verify the manufacturer's claims prior to purchasing a filter. The National Sanitation Foundation is an independent testing agency that evaluates and certifies the performance of filtering devices.
- Install a shower filter system.
- Replace faucets if identified as the source of lead.
- Replace pipes.
- Use bottled water. Since not all bottled water is lead-free, check the label on your water. The water contains no lead if the Pb (lead) content is listed as zero.
- Warm or hot tap water is likely to contain more lead; use only cold water for preparing baby formula, drinking and cooking.
- Replace garden hoses with lead-free alternatives.

STEP TWO: If you brought it home and it contains lead, get rid of it

It is an understandable concern that the list of products that contain lead seems never-ending. However, when the exercise is complete and the dangerous items have been removed, it is far less likely that you will repeat buying dangerous lead-containing products. In other words, this process will also hone your consumer skills.

Getting rid of items that you discover contain lead takes some thoughtfulness. Having a garage sale to sell items to families who are unaware that the products contain lead defeats the purpose, as does tossing the items in the trash where they will ultimately contaminate the landfill and the lead will leach its way back into the ecological cycle. Take the high road and resist the attempt to dump it on others or in the garbage. Identifying which things need to go is the easy part. Ironically, the step of getting rid of lead-endowed items you do not want in your house may be the bigger challenge. Replace those things that must be replaced. When it comes to non-necessity items such as toys, enjoy the purge and relish the physical and psychological space you have created in your life. Again, resist the urge to give items to Goodwill just to be redistributed amongst less privileged children. Look out for them by *not* donating your unwanted items.

Deciding what to test

Lead from toys and household objects is dangerous when it is chewed or sucked on, or when touched and then transferred from hand to mouth. Adults and older children put their hands in their mouths or suck and chew on things less often than babies and small children. A little observation will go a long way over the next few weeks as you work your way through the second step in eliminating and reducing lead exposure from your family's routines and activities. An excellent place to begin is by reading the Centers for Disease Control and Prevention's recall lists at http://www.cdc.gov/nceh/lead/Recalls/allhazards.htm. The lists will not only alert you to any items that can be removed immediately, they will also give you a sense of what kinds of items contain lead and how lead is used in manufacturing. Also, read through the list of potential lead sources (see appendix 3), for common household items, and check back through any notes you may have made in the process of reading the previous chapters of this book.

Items at risk of containing lead may not be evident immediately, but your awareness will grow as you work through the process. Test things as you recognize them as a risk. In the meantime, if you eat off them, test them. If your baby mouths them, test them. If you or your children handle them, test them.

Test kits

Lead testing kits currently available for purchase at home centers, hardware stores and online are typically designed to detect surface lead but are not intended to identify specific lead levels. They are limited in their ability to reveal lead embedded below the surface, under a layer of protective or decorative coating. Thus, obtaining an accurate reading of lead content is more challenging on objects that may contain lead in their composite materials or in the paints and glazes they have been finished with. Also, since the presence of lead is indicated by a color change, the results can be affected by pigments used in the production of these products. Even though the results from these tests are not as accurate as those obtained from a professional lab, they can be useful tools to begin the process of identifying items containing lead. Turn to appendix 2 for a list of lead test kits that received a passing grade from the US Consumer Report.

Sampling technique

The way you test the glaze on your dishes will vary from how you test the paint on your child's pencil. Toys and other objects made of wood and vinyl and decorated with paint or enamel will need to be tested differently than those made of metal or containing lead solder, which may be coated with another substance. Kits that employ swabs or are designed expressly for certain types of lead surfaces are helpful. Follow the specific instructions carefully. But generally, for painted wood and vinyl, test the painted surface by cutting into the paint with a sharp blade or scratching up the surface of the vinyl. Take your sample from this exposed area. For painted metal, metal parts or soldered components you will need to actually cut through any outside layer to access the metal. Ensure that any cuts made will not create a hazardous edge, and that the cut is in an inconspicuous place. Be sure to write each tested item in the lead inventory log in appendix 1, with the date and method of testing and the results. This will be important information for creating your response plan.

Options for testing

Hiring a company to come and test your home and everything in it is an option. There are several considerations in hiring someone to do this for you, the expense being the obvious one. Another drawback is that the window of testing is limited to a snapshot in time. Using a home testing kit, although you must do your homework and choose a reliable and accurate product, allows for ongoing vigilance as purchases are made and gifts are received over weeks and months.

Interpretation of results

There is no safe level of lead, so all readings should be heeded as a warning to eliminate the source or avoid exposure. Pay attention to the sensitivity of your kit. Some kits do not accurately read lead levels below ten or fifteen micrograms. These are very high levels and items showing lead above ten micrograms should be removed immediately. Swabs which identify the presence of lead without specifying the lead level should be a catalyst for action no matter that you lack a specific measurement.

Developing a response plan

As toys and household items are identified, you should not delay in removing them to an area of the house or garage with limited access while you finish testing and create a plan for getting rid of them. There is no logic in allowing a child to keep playing with a toy or for you to keep wearing a chain that contains lead while you decide what to do with it. Move it to the garage or secured storage *now.* Plan on how to safely and responsibly get rid of it later.

At the beginning of the book, we talked about the ripple your personal action would create as you moved through this process of learning and becoming empowered. If you have an expensive toy or item that tests as containing lead, consider returning it to the store where you bought it. If you have the bill, or a credit card statement showing the purchase, so much the better. If not, do not be optimistic about getting a refund or credit. Your objective should be to give the object back to the store so that they take responsibility for it, not to recoup money that was spent in what is essentially a buyer-beware world. Ask for the manager and be respectful and polite. Remember, the individuals you are speaking to may ethically and morally have a responsibility, but ultimately they are paid employees who know less about lead and its effects than you do. Take the book if you like and show the manager your inventory. Explain how you discovered the product you assumed was safe is putting you and your family at risk. If you do not get to see a manager, or it is a small-ticket item, give it back to the clerk at the return counter. Let them know why you are returning it and leave it with them to deal with.

Alternatively, write a brief letter to the company and mail the item back to them. Again, your main objective is to safely and responsibly remove the item from your home. Engaging the activist in you is secondary and something you can pursue later—when your house is lead-free!

STEP THREE: Check surfaces, indoors and out

Now the water you drink and wash with is free of lead. Your home and work areas have had items that contain lead removed. The third stage of lead-proofing yourself and your family is to assess surfaces, indoors and out. By this we mean the paint on your walls, the finishes on your furniture, the dust on your shelving, and the soil in your yard.

List the sites for testing

Once again, scan over the recall lists with a focus on painted or clear-coated furniture surfaces. Normal household dust typically contains lead as a result of interior paint that contains lead, renovations in a house that contains lead paint, or vicinity to a lead source such as a lead smelter or industrial site where lead is being sanded, e.g., a bridge undergoing repainting, a race track, shooting range, etc.

For now, the focus will be on your own house and yard. Inside, go room by room, leaving rooms least frequented until last. The garage, carport, shed, and porch areas are also important to check. In the yard, walk about noting exposed soil or sand, especially near the house, fence and outbuildings. Patches of exposed dirt under swing sets or play equipment should be included on the list and made a testing priority if they are frequently accessed by gardeners, children or pets.

List the indoor rooms and areas you will test:

_____   _____

_____   _____

_____   _____

_____   _____

_____   _____

_____   _____

_____   _____

With your rooms and areas identified, go back and prioritize. Number according to the most urgent and important to test. Places where your family spends the most time will have the highest priority; who uses them and how much contact they have with the various surfaces are factors in how you prioritize. Having a sense of which sources are most critical will assist you in developing your response plan later.

Now repeat this process for your outdoor areas:

_____   _____

_____   _____

_____   _____

_____   _____

_____   _____

_____   _____

_____   _____

Sampling technique

Painted or varnished surfaces on walls or furniture:

Begin by making sure that the painted area you wish to test is clean and dry. If necessary, use a household cleaner, rinsing and drying well. Choose a discreet area of the wall or furniture where the test area will not be obvious. Using a sharp blade, remove a small v-shaped notch, about three to five millimeters in length (3/32 to 3/16 inch), being sure to go deep enough into multiple layers of paint to expose all of them.

Dust:

A sample of dust can be swabbed in place or collected using a baby-wipe. Samples can be placed in sealable plastic sandwich bags and labeled. Be sure that the surface the dust has landed on is negative for lead so that your results can be interpreted and responded to correctly.

Soil and sand:

Generally, a soil or sand sample is collected and sent to a lab for analysis. Depending on who is testing it, the methodology for sample collection will change slightly. Basically though, it involves nothing more than putting a few scoops of soil from the region of testing into the container or bag supplied in the test kit. The scoop or shovel needs to be made of plastic or a non-reactive metal and should be clean. The sample should be obtained from the top ten to fifteen centimeters (four to six inches) for gardens, one to four centimeters (one-half to two inches) for children's play areas; not deeper. Gloves are recommended. Collect up to a dozen sub-samples from one area, mix them in a bucket and then draw one final sample from the mix. About one cup is all that a lab requires for analysis. Repeat for each yard area that is of concern, creating a map of the yard and marking where each numbered sample was drawn from. Alternatively, or additionally, you can put small labeled stakes in the ground, according to your circumstance. Record each test and related information in the inventory found in the appendix.

Options for testing

The initial stage for checking the dust and surfaces in your home can be completed by carefully following instructions on a home lead test kit. The most reliable way to test soil or sand, however, is to take collected samples to a provincially or state licensed lab or a locally offered testing service. Some counties and municipalities run testing programs for area residents.

Interpretation of results

Indoors:

Any reading of lead in dust or paint surfaces is a cause for concern and a call for action. Paint with lead that is chipping or peeling is obviously a bigger concern than that which is in good repair. Also consider who comes in contact with it and how. Contaminated clear coat on a crib that a toddler chews on, or a window that opens and closes often and generates a steady supply of leaded paint dust, need to be addressed with urgency. Antique furniture with leaded varnish, intact, in a living room that is rarely entered by adults and never by children, is a low priority. High lead levels in everyday dust, however, may warrant further investigation as to the source.

Outdoors:

Soils that contain lead levels of 100 parts per million or higher should not be used for gardening. Children and pets should not have access to garden areas where there is any measurable lead identified.

Developing a response plan

Indoors:

Once dangerous furniture items have been removed, you will need to ascertain what measures are warranted with regard to any lead-containing paint. Lead abatement should strictly be done by professionals. General or routine dust removal calls for vacuuming with HEPA filter equipment or a closed system with care taken not to stir up or re-circulate lead-containing dust. Vacuuming should be followed by wet-wiping furniture surfaces. Most importantly, however, if your dust contains lead, your response plan should include determining whether the source of the lead is in your home and can be removed, or from a remote source which may require engaging your local authorities in a resolution.

Outdoors:

There are a number of ways to address lead-contaminated soil. If you opt to dig out the soil and remove it from the yard completely, be aware that there are strict regulations that must be adhered to depending on the area where you live. Do not violate these regulations during disposal of your contaminated soil. As an alternative to removal, you could opt to make the lead unavailable to plants by raising the soil pH. This is done by adding healthy compost material to the soil and possibly adding a layer of sod. You could also cover the contaminated soil with fresh soil and then a ground cover. It is strongly recommended that you do not leave soil bare where it has been tested as containing lead.

NOTES

CHAPTER 12

BODY BURDEN: GETTING THE LEAD OUT

We have left the removal of past lead accumulations and other heavy metals to the final chapter for a reason: there would be no point in beginning a process of removing metals from the body if a steady stream of new toxins was simply taking their place.

If you have now completed the three steps outlined in the inventory, you and your family have clean, lead free water to drink and wash with. Toys and household items that were lead sources have been banished to the garage, even if you have not quite finished going through and disposing of them safely. You have covered any lead-contaminated soil or sand in your yard and identified and eliminated the source of lead that was making everyday house dust toxic. As well, you have stopped bringing lead home from work on your clothing, shoes and hair. If you had obtained a blood test at the start of your household lead intervention, that would have told you how much lead was regularly entering your body. If a few months have passed, having your blood lead level retested is a way to measure your success at removing the lead sources.

When it comes to the removal of lead that has accumulated in your body over time, there are many approaches. Each person's state of health, age, metabolism, biology and toxic load must be taken into account when deciding how best to approach this. Therefore, it is especially important that you locate a doctor in your area who understands heavy metal toxicity and who can guide you through a process that is safe and effective for you. Medical supervision is imperative while removing lead and other toxins from your body. Removal that is too invasive or aggressive can be dangerous. Just as there are risks in leaving lead in the body, there are risks with removing it. These are concerns that you will need to discuss with your doctor.

Natural Approaches

There is a growing list of alternative lead removal methods. Options range from far infrared saunas and clay footbaths, to herbal preparations that use the synergistic effect of cilantro and chlorella. Cilantro, chlorella and garlic are three commonly used natural products.

Cilantro, also known as Chinese parsley and coriander, is an herb used commonly in Mexican, Middle Eastern and African cooking, as well as in folk medicine. It is abundant in chlorophyll, contains vitamins C and A, as well as calcium and niacin. Cilantro has been shown to suppress lead deposition and lead-induced kidney damage in mice.[139] Cilantro is said to stimulate the body's mechanism for heavy metal removal. A study by the Heart Disease Research Foundation indicated that cilantro has the ability to remove heavy metals from the human system. This research reported that once the heavy metals were removed using cilantro, the patients were less susceptible to colds, flu and Herpes outbreaks.[140] A Japanese study found that cilantro has the ability to remove heavy metals from the body in about two weeks. To obtain its healing maximal effects, cilantro must be eaten fresh.[141]

Chlorella is a type of green, fresh water, one-cell algae that has been reported to be very effective in eliminating heavy metals from bones, connective tissue, muscles, ligaments, the brain and intestinal wall. Chlorella contains more chlorophyll per gram than any other plant. Dehydrated chlorella powder contains over fifty percent protein and it is a significant provider of beta-carotene, RNA and vitamin B12. Chlorella is also a source of vitamin C, vitamins B1, B2, B3, B5, B6, folic acid and biotin. A study conducted on lead-poisoned mice showed that treatment with chlorella significantly reduced lead levels in blood and tissue.[142]

Garlic is a natural detoxifier. According to an article from *Better Nutrition,* garlic aids the liver in reducing levels of lead and other poisons. It increases the activity of a number of liver enzymes such as glutathione-S-transferase and cytochrome P450. Researchers discovered that garlic not only plays a role in lead poisoning prevention but it diminishes symptoms of lead poisoning as well.[143] Garlic has been shown to reduce lead levels in animals. High lead levels in animals dramatically decrease after being fed garlic cloves. Because of garlic's detoxification properties, it can be helpful in ensuring that the body is doing the best possible job getting rid of poisons it encounters.

Medical Approaches

Currently available "mainstream" methods used to decrease the lead body burden involve some form of chelation, a process in which a chelating agent binds with lead that resides in soft tissues, thus helping with excretion. The word chelation comes from a Greek word "chele" that means to claw. The US Department of Health and Human Services lists four chelating agents that are in use today: DMPS, D pennicilamine, BAL, and EDTA.

DMPS, also known under the name of 2,3-dimercaptosuccinic acid, succimer or Chemet, is the most commonly prescribed chelating agent used to treat lead poisoning. Doctors prefer this medication because it can be administered orally on an outpatient basis and compared with other chelating agents, it removes less of the wanted zinc, iron, calcium, manganese and copper. It is approved for use with children and adults. Like other chelating agents it binds with lead and together they are excreted in the urine. DMPS is available as a capsule. In some cases, it can be taken concurrently with iron. It has a bad smell and taste so to make it easier to administer it can be sprinkled on food, especially something sweet tasting like ice cream or pudding.

DMPS may cause adverse side effects such as elevated liver enzymes, susceptibility to infection, anorexia, nausea, vomiting, fatigue and skin rash.

D penicillamine, also called Cuprimine, binds with organic lead and increases the amount of excreted lead via urine. Like DMPS, it is administered orally. The mechanism of how this chelator works is scientifically uncertain, thus it has not been approved by the US Food and Drug Administration to be administered to pregnant women or children. The process of removing lead from the body using this method can take up to several months. D penicillamine can be obtained in capsules or tablets. It can be swallowed by itself or mixed with food or drink.

Side effects may include anorexia, nausea, vomiting, fever, skin rash, decreased white cells, low platelets, high levels of eosinophils in the blood, hemolytic anemia, Stevens-Johnson syndrome (a potentially deadly skin disease), kidney toxicity and an excess of serum proteins in the urine. It is critical that the environmental lead source is eliminated, as the rate of lead absorption increases when taking this medication.

BAL, also known as Anti-Lewisite and Dimercaprol, is most commonly used while the renal function is compromised, in cases of asymptomatic and symptomatic high lead levels and in acute brain toxicity. It is administered intravenously as a ten percent solution in oil. Lead is excreted via fecal matter, bile and urine.

Adverse effects of this medication include fever, hypertension, rapid heartbeat, anxiety, headache, nausea, vomiting, increased excretions and abdominal pain. Its use is contraindicated for pregnant women, for individuals with liver failure, glucose-6-phosphate dehydrogenize deficiency, and those with a history of allergy to peanut oil.

EDTA or CANA2-EDTA is a synthetic amino acid. It works by increasing renal lead excretion. As a treatment for lead poisoning, it was first introduced in the United States in 1948. It is administered intravenously and is approved for adults and children. As too much lead becomes mobilized and recycled in the blood stream while taking EDTA alone, it is usually taken concurrently with BAL. Numerous adverse effects have been reported. They include fever, chills, thirst, rash, muscle pains and cardiac arrhythmia. Unfortunately, EDTA chelates not only lead but also zinc and cadmium. Precautions must be taken in persons with low zinc levels and those with occupational cadmium exposure.

The intention of this book is not to recommend any particular method or approach, as clearly that is the domain of the medical profession. We do recommend, however, that you do your homework, research your options and then agree upon a plan with your doctor or naturopath. Obviously, an accumulation of lead that took decades cannot be removed in a day or a week. The ultimate goal is to build the healthiest system possible so removing lead should be but one step in restoring your overall health.

Final Thoughts

It is not a fad or a theory that lead causes damage to the human body and brain. It creates more types of damage, earlier and more often than was ever thought before. We now have more than a generation of children with sometimes invisible but serious brain damage to show for our casual attitude toward lead. We know that the specific brain damage that lead causes manifests itself as learning disabilities, ADHD, low IQ and delinquent behavior. As scientists emerge from their research silos and cross-reference their findings, there is a rapidly growing body of evidence that in partnership with mercury, lead is an underlying causal factor of autism. The link between heavy metals and autoimmune disease has been established.

As you reach the end of this book, you will realize that it is not the end of your journey. Safeguarding against lead and its harmful effects will be an ongoing commitment. It is, however, time to pause and commend yourself. You have taken steps to break a cycle that is on a dangerous trajectory. You now have the knowledge and the resources to minimize accidental and daily lead exposure and to stop the epidemic of damage that so many have resigned themselves to believing is simply the cost of living in a modern world.

APPENDIX 1

LEAD INVENTORIES

STEP ONE INVENTORY

Sample No.	Source	Date tested	Test/Lab used	LEAD pp/ml	Priority hi med lo	Response plan	Done ☑
e.g., SAMPLE 1	Kitchen faucet: first draw-cold	Jan 7/09	Municipal Testing	6.0	high	John will arrange for installation of under counter water filter by Jan 30/08 Cost: $ 199.99	✓
e.g., SAMPLE 2	Kitchen faucet: flush - cold	Jan 7/09	Fraser Health Authority	2.0	high	John will arrange for installation of under counter water filter by Jan 30/08 Cost: $ 199.99	✓
e.g., SAMPLE 3	Kitchen faucet: hot	Jan 7/09	Fraser Health Authority	12.0	high	John will arrange for installation of under counter water filter by Jan 30/08 Cost: $ 199.99	✓

Sample No.	Source		Date tested	Test/Lab used	LEAD pp/ml	Priority hi med lo	Response plan		Done ☑

STEP TWO INVENTORY

Source	Date tested	Test/Lab used	LEAD present	Priority	Response plan	Done ☑
e.g.,: dinner plates	Feb 5/09	LEADcheck Kit	YES	High	Move dishes to sealed box in garage then return to department store.	✔ To-do

Source	Date tested	Test/Lab used	LEAD present	Priority	Response plan	Done ☑

STEP THREE INVENTORY

Source	Date tested	Test/Lab used	LEAD present	Priority	Response plan	Done ☑
e.g., front garden	Mar3/09	Municipal soil testing service	YES	medium	John will replace contaminated soil and plant Creeping Thyme as ground cover.	✔

Source	Date tested	Test/Lab used	LEAD present	Priority	Response plan	Done ☑

APPENDIX 2

TESTING PRODUCTS

Water Testing

Test name	Retail Price	Features
WATERSAFE	$ 10.00	one-step test detects dissolved lead levels below 15 parts per billion gives results in 10 minutes
LEAD CHECK AQUA	$ 17.00	detects dissolved lead levels above 15 parts per billion takes 10 to 15 minutes from start to finish
LEAD INSPECTOR	$ 13.00	colors on the chart show approximate lead levels from 1 to higher than 50 parts per million
COLE-PALMER LEAD TEST for WATER SUPPLIES	$ 81.00 to $ 88.00	test strip is inserted into a sample and then treated with a reactive dye to determine presence of lead three sensitivity levels: 1 to 4 parts per million, 15 parts per million or higher, and 250 to 750 parts per billion

General Lead Testing

Test name	Retail Price	Features	Use
HOMAX LEAD CHECK	$ 8.00	cigarette-shaped swabs turn pink when lead is present, easy to use	test the presence of accessible lead in household items such as toys, ceramic dishware, vinyl, or plastic
LEAD CHECK HOUSEHOLD LEAD TEST KIT	$19.00	cigarette shaped swabs turn pink when lead is present easy to use	test the presence of accessible lead in household items such as toys, ceramic dishware, vinyl, or plastic
LEAD INSPECTOR	$ 13.00	swabs turn yellow, brown, gray, or black if lead is detected	test household items such as toys, jewelry, ceramics, vinyl, or plastic; used to test soil, water, paint and dust

Adapted from ConsumerReports.org

APPENDIX 3

POSSIBLE SOURCES OF LEAD

ALLOYS

- brass
- bronze
- pewter
- terne plating

ART AND HOBBY MATERIALS

- ceramic dyes and glazes
- crayons and chalk
- glass paint
- imported craft items (painted buttons, etc)
- lines for fishing
- paints—especially with names "Flake White" and "Lead White"
- solder for jewelry making, lead lighting, etc
- stained glass came
- statuary
- t-shirt transfers

BUILDINGS AND STRUCTURES

- bathroom or shower floors
- brass and bronze alloys for plumbing valves or fixtures
- bronze and brass plaques
- cable sheathing for telephone and power cables
- caulking
- ceramic tiles
- damp-proof building structures
- earthquake dampening materials
- fireplace surrounds
- fountain fittings
- lead head roof nails and lead washers for galvanized screws used on roofing iron
- lead-light such as used on kitchen cupboards
- lead solder for plumbing

- lighting assemblies
- old gas and water pipes
- old glazing putty
- paint
- pewter
- porcelain bathtubs
- PVC insulation
- red lead as a sealant on the back of old linoleum
- roofing cover
- sheet lead flashing
- solder on guttering
- soldered copper pipes
- sound insulation
- submersible pump in wells
- water header tanks in the ceiling space
- white lead and linseed oil based putty
- wrought iron

CARS

- batteries
- car seat fabric
- leaded gasoline (race, collector cars)
- metal joinery
- moulding
- solder
- wheel balance weights
- wheel bearings

CONSUMABLES

- ayurvedic medicines
- calcium supplements
- candy
- chocolate
- cigarettes
- diarrhea remedies that contain attapulgite clay

- eggs from poultry housed on contaminated soil
- folk remedies (see appendix 4)
- food grown on land contaminated by lead fall-out (industry or traffic) or by lead contaminated super-phosphate, trace metal fertilizers or sewage sludge
- fresh fruit and vegetables (natural lead levels can be especially high in spinach and silver-beet)
- game meat
- imported candy
- imported canned food
- imported spices and seasoning
- raisins
- sweetener in older medicine
- water
- waterfowl
- wine

COSMETICS

- hair color restorer treatments
- henna
- imported eye cosmetics
- imported cosmetics such as kohl
- powder, baby talcum and baby creams
- some 'progressive' hair dyes
- some lipstick

ENVIRONMENTAL SOURCES

- ash and emissions from burning painted wood
- ash and emissions from coal-burning
- ash and emissions from wood-burning
- dust from demolition of lead shot production towers, buildings, bridges, and plants
- emissions from metallurgical works and metal heat treating works
- erosion of lead ore bodies

- human (and animal) cremation (95% of lead is stored in bones)
- soil and dust near lead industries, roadways, lead-painted houses
- volcanic eruptions
- waste and emissions from ferrous and non-ferrous foundries
- waste and emissions from lead and silver and zinc mines and smelters

FOOD AND DRINK CONTAINERS

- bronze dishes
- ceramics
- glass
- hot beverage machine parts such as in cappuccino makers, hot water urns
- imported food can solder
- leaded crystal
- leaded decals (transfers) on drinking glasses
- lead foil tops covering the corks of old wine bottles
- lead shot weighted beverage hygrometers
- pewter dishes
- polyethylene food-wrapping film
- old crockery
- old cutlery
- old lead-lined pots and pans
- old moonshine made in stills made from car radiators, lead pipes, etc
- polishing agent for luster finish marble chopping boards
- pottery
- samovars
- water tank lining on some tanks

INDUSTRIAL USES

- acid plants
- cable trunking, cabling and wire

- catalysts
- chemical treatment baths
- electrical conduit
- electronics
- explosives
- glass (decorative, optical, ophthalmic, electrical, radiation protection)
- lead sheet (flashing, roofing, cladding)
- lead wool
- lubricants
- pigments
- plastic insulation on electrical wiring
- plastic resins
- PVC
- solder for electronics and appliances
- soundproofing
- stabilizers
- storage batteries
- storage vessels

INKS, DYES AND PRINTING

- cheap color newspaper
- fabrics
- leather tanning compounds
- packaging
- old printing
- older typeset and plates
- roller coating, flexographic and screen inks for packaging

PAINT

- accessories such as buttons and snaps
- aircraft and spacecraft
- appliances
- car and marine primers and topcoats
- farm and other equipment

- lead powder in corrosion-resistant paint
- metal furniture
- mirror backing
- painting (artists' paints)
- primers and industrial paints
- sign and road-marking paints
- steel or iron primer
- wood furniture

PLASTICS AND CHEMICALS

- catalysts
- compounds for cloud-making
- compounds in old match-heads
- heat stabilizers, e.g. in PVC
- lead compounds in plastic resins
- lead compounds in rubber manufacture
- lead oxide in glassmaking
- lead pigmented colored glass
- lubricants
- PVC building profiles
- PVC cladding
- PVC coated electrical cable e.g. Christmas light wires etc
- PVC coated wire for fences, coat hangers, clothes horses
- PVC flexible extrusion including wall plugs, curtain rods, insulation, furniture trim
- PVC flooring
- PVC footwear
- PVC guttering
- PVC hose including food and beverage hose
- PVC mini-blinds
- PVC mouldings
- PVC piping and trunking such as components for hydroponics
- PVC solar tubing for heating swimming pools
- PVC unsupported film and sheet such as stationery (folders), packaging, hospital bed sheeting, clothing, belting

- PVC vinyl coated fabrics such as seating, clothing, awnings, signs
- PVC window profiles
- old dry cleaning fluids
- pigments
- tile and other glazing compounds

PLUMBING

- bath and toilet ceramics
- brass fittings and fixtures
- older water tank solder
- non-potable PVC piping
- PVC
- solder

PRODUCT PACKAGING

- anticorrosive liners for storage drums
- certain plastics
- tubing

RADIATION SHIELDING

- home radon liners
- VDU and TV screen
- lead powder
- sheet lead for radiation shielding including aprons and lead vests for dentists, radiologists, etc

SPORTS AND HOBBIES see chapter 2

TRANSPORT AND FUEL APPLICATIONS

- auto body solder for panel beating (burning and grinding)
- aviation fuel for spark ignition non-jet engines
- boat ballast

- cable sheathing on marine vessel cables
- lead-acid batteries
- marine paint
- older cars and motorcycles
- older boats
- pendulum weights for seat belts
- propeller aircraft
- PVC body side moulding and mud flaps, etc
- PVC flexible bumper strip
- PVC oil and air filters
- PVC in vehicle interiors e.g. mats
- radiator solder
- ship keels
- sump-oil contaminated sawdust
- tetra alkyl lead octane enhancer for automotive and motor-mower fuels
- terne plated metal in fuel tank lining
- train brake pads
- wheel balancing lead weights
- weights for boats' and ships' ballast

OTHER

- accessories such as key chains
- artificial Christmas trees
- ashtrays
- baby bibs
- balance for whip handles
- candles with a leaded metal core wick
- chalk
- children's clothes
- Christmas decorations
- Christmas lights
- crayons
- curtain weights
- diving weights
- door stops

- electronic lead solder in appliances and computers
- electronics
- fertilizers such as lead arsenate (in the past used as a pesticide mainly on apples and tobacco)
- furniture trim (PVC bumper strips)
- garden hoses
- inexpensive and toy jewelry
- lamp stands
- lead coffins and other funerary items
- lead weights for milking teats in milking machines
- lead weights in non-tip children's cups
- lunchboxes
- jewelry (lead, pewter, brass, bronze)
- marble polish
- moulding on shoes
- old metal toothpaste tubes
- paperweights
- piano keys
- plastic insulation on telephone wiring
- raingear
- security seals such as on gas meters
- storage batteries (lead-acid batteries)
- toys
- toy soldiers and other models
- t-shirt transfers
- vinyl coated fabrics
- umbrellas
- used motor oil for weed suppression
- weighted crayfish traps and fishing nets
- weights for analytical instruments
- weights for go karts
- weights for yacht keels
- weights in wool presses
- weights to make "sleep eyes" in dolls
- wooden and lead components in French game

Sources: Environmental Protection Authority
Oregon Department of Human Services
The Lead Group of Australia

APPENDIX 4

TRADITIONAL REMEDIES AND COSMETICS

Product Name	Region of Origin What it Looks Like	Lead Content	Used For
Albayalde or Albayaidle	Mexico and Central America	93%	upset stomach, apathy, lethargy
Alarcon, Azarcon, Coral, Luiga, Maria Luisa, or Rueda	Mexico bright orange powder	95%	upset stomach constipation, diarrhea, vomiting, teething powder
Alkohl	Middle East	85%	topical preparation applied to umbilical stump
Al Murrah	Saudi Arabia		colic, upset stomach, diarrhea
Anzroot	Middle East		stomach flu
Ba-Baw-San	China	1000 mg/g	colic pain, hyperactivity and nightmares in children
Bala Goli	Asia/India black bean		upset stomach
Bint Al Zahab, Bint or Bent Dahab	Iran, Oman, Saudi Arabia, India ground rock	98%	diarrhea, colic, constipation, and general neonatal use

Product Name	Region of Origin What it Looks Like	Lead Content	Used For
Bokhoor (Noqd)	Saudi Arabia Practice of burning wood and lead sulphide to produce fumes.		used to calm infants
Cebagin	Middle East	51%	teething powder
Chuifong Tokuwan, Black Pearls or Miracle Herb	Asia herbal mixture		arthritis
Cordyceps	China	414-20,000 ug/g	hypertension, diabetes, bleeding
Deshi Dewa	Asia, India	12%	infertility
Farouk	Saudi Arabia		teething powder
Ghasard	India brown powder	2%	digestion aid
Greta	Mexico bright orange powder	97%	upset stomach, constipation, diarrhea, vomiting, teething powder
Hai Ge Fen	China clamshell powder	22.5%	gastrointestinal ailments

Product Name	Region of Origin What it Looks Like	Lead Content	Used For
Jin Bu Huan	China		pain relieve
Kandu	Asia/India red powder		upset stomach
Kohl, Alkohl or Saoott	Africa, Asia, India, Pakistan, Middle East	Up to 86%	eye cosmetic, astringent for eye injuries, applied to umbilical stump, teething powder
Kushta	India/Pakistan	73%	heart, brain, liver, and stomach disease, aphrodisiac
Litargirio	Dominican Republic powder	79%	foot fungus
Mahayogaray gugullu	India tonic		high blood pressure
Pay-loo-ah	Laos, Vietnam red powder	90%	fever, rash
Po Ying Tan	China		minor ailments in children
Santrinj	Saudi Arabia amorphous red powder	98%	teething powder, gum boils

Product Name	Region of Origin What it Looks Like	Lead Content	Used For
Surma	India black powder		cosmetics, teething powder
Tibetan herbal vitamin	Tibet		to strengthen the brain
Traditional Saudi Medicine	Saudi Arabia orange powder		teething, diarrhea

ENDNOTES

1   Lewis, J. (1985). Lead poisoning: historical perspective. *EPA Journal* on line: http://www.epa.gov/history/topics/perspect/lead.htm.

2   Ibid.

3   Wedeen, R. P. (1984). *Poison in the Pot. The Legacy of Lead.* Southern Illinois University Press: Carbondaly & Edwardsville.

4   Ibid.

5   Lewis, J. (1985). Lead poisoning: historical perspective. *EPA Journal* on line: http://www.epa.gov/history/topics/perspect/lead.htm.

6   Oliver, P. (1911). A lecture on lead poisoning and the race. Quoted in J. S. Lin-Fu, (1980), Lead poisoning and undue lead exposure in children: history and current status. In H. L. Needleman, (Eds.), *Low Level Lead Exposure: The Clinical Implications of Current Research*, Raven Press, New York, NY.

7   Dickens, C. (n.d.) The uncommercial traveler. *The Works of Charles Dickens in Thirty Volumes.* New York: P. F. Collier & Son.

8   *Mysteries of Canada: The Franklin Expedition.* Retrieved January 12, 2007 from http://www.mysteriesofcanada.com/Nunavut/franklin.htm.

9   Lin-Fu, J. S. (1980). Lead poisoning and undue lead exposure in children: history and current status. In H. L. Needleman, (Eds.), *Low Level Lead Exposure: The Clinical Implications of Current Research*, Raven Press, New York, NY.

10   Ruddock, J. C. (1924). Lead poisoning in children, *Journal of the American Medical Association, 83*, 1682-4.

11   Lin-Fu, J. S. (1980). Lead poisoning and undue lead exposure in children: history and current status. In H. L. Needleman, (Eds.), *Low Level Lead Exposure: The Clinical Implications of Current Research*, Raven Press, New York, NY.

12   Ibid.

13   Rothenberg, S.J., & Rothenberg, J.C. (2005). Testing the Dose-Response Specification in Epidemiology. Public Health and Policy Consequences for Lead. *Environmental Health Perspectives, 113(9).*

14   Canfield, R. L., Henderson, C. R., Cory-Slechta, D. A., Cox, C., Jusko, T. A., & Lanphear, P. B. (2003). Intellectual impairment in children with blood-lead concentrations below 10 micrograms per decilitre. *New England Journal of Medicine, 384,* 1517-1526.

15 Cincinnati Children's Hospital Medical Center. (n.d.). *History of Lead Advertising.* Retrieved September 15, 2008 from http://www.cincinnatichildrens.org/research/project/enviro/hazard/lead.

16 Gulson, B.L. (2000). "Revision of estimates of skeletal contribution to blood during pregnancy and postpartum period." Journal of Laboratory and Clinical Medicine, 136, 250–251.

17 Gulson, B.L., Jameson, C.W., Mahaffey, K.R., Mizon, K.J., Patison, N., & Law, A.J. (1998). "Relationships of lead in breast milk to lead in blood, urine, and diet of the infant and mother." Environmental Health Perspectives, 106, 667– 674.

18 Chocolate Manufacturers Association. (2005). A Characterization of Lead in Chocolate Products.

19 American Environmental Safety Institute. (May 2002). Lead in Chocolate: The Impact on Children's Health. Fact Sheet.

20 Haas, E.M., Levin, B. (2006). Staying Healthy with Nutrition the Complete Guide to Diet and Nutritional Medicine. California: Celestial Arts.

21 Get the Lead Out. Retrieved September 19, 2008 from http://www.fjta.org/docs/GetLeadOut.pdf.

22 Ibid.

23 Centers for Disease Control and Prevention. Department of Health and Human Services. Lead Recalls. Retrieved May 24, 2008 from http://www.cdc.gov/nceh/lead/Recalls/default.htm.

24 Martha Mendoza Associated Press. (2007). "Are Lunch Boxes a Health Danger?" Retrieved March 14, 2008 from http://findarticles.com/p/articles/mi_qn4188/is_/ai_n18623484.

25   Center for Environmental Health (2007). Legal Action Forces Wal-Mart to Pull Lead Tainted Baby Bibs in Three States. Retrieved November 15, 2008 from http://www.ceh.org/index. php?option=com_content&task=view&id=176&Itemid=166.

26   National Safety Council. (1996). "CPSC Finds Lead Poisoning Hazard for Young Children in Imported Vinyl Miniblinds." Retrieved April 24, 2008 from http://www.nsc.org/resources/ issues/alerts/lead_mini_blinds.aspx.

27   Maas, R.P., Patch, S.C, Pandolfo, T.J., Druhan, J.L., & Gandy, N.F. (2005). Artificial Christmas trees: how real are the lead exposure risks? Bulletin of Environmental Contamination and Toxicology, 7(3) 437-44.

28   Lead Poisoning Prevention. (n.d). Retrieved January 03, 2008 from http://orgs.unca.edu/eqi/lpp/where.html#chalk.

29   Prismark Partners LLC. (2002). "Lead Free Electronic Assembly: How Will This Unfold?" Retrieved January 03, 2008 from http://www.amd.com.cn/CHCN/assets/content_type/ DownloadableAssets/2002_June_17_Prismark_.pdf.

30   The Campaign for Safe Cosmetics. (2007). "A Poison Kiss: The Problem of Lead in Lipstick." Retrieved January 17, 2008 from www.safecosmetics.org.

31   Gittleman, J.L., Engelgau, M.M., Shaw, J., et.al. (1994). "Lead poisoning among battery reclamation workers in Alabama." Journal of Occupational Medicine, 36, 526-32.

32   Environmental Working Group. (2001). "Lead in Outdoor Firing Ranges." Retrieved April 24, 2008 from www.ewg.org/ reports/poisonouspasttime.

33   Natale Servino. "NASCAR Goes Green?" Earth Island Journal. Retrieved February 03, 2008 from http://www.earthisland.org/eijournal/new_articles. cfm?articleID=981&journalID=84.

34   Jim Cressman. "Leaded fuel ban could nix racing." Sun Media, January 23, 2008.

35   Lead Poisoning Prevention Program, "Possible Sources of Lead Exposure." Retrieved February 14, 2007 from www. healthoregon.org/lead.

36   US Department of Health and Human Services. (2007). Toxicological Profile for Lead.

37   Chamberlain, A.C., Heard, M.J., Little, P., Newton, D., Wells, A.C., & Wiffen, R.D. (1978). AERE-R 9198. Oxon, UK: Harwell.

38   Yip, Y.K. (1981). "Partial purification and characterization of human (immune) interferon." The Proceedings of the National Academy of Sciences USA, 78, 1601-1605.

39   Johnson, N.E., & Tenuta, K. (1979). "Diets and blood leads of children who practice pica." Environmental Research 18, 369–376.

40   Bellinger, D., Leviton, A., Waternaux, C., Needleman, H.L., & Rabinowitz, M. (1987). "Longitudinal analyses of prenatal and postnatal lead exposure and early cognitive development." New England Journal of Medicine, 316, 1037-43.

41   US Department of Health and Human Services. (2007). Toxicological Profile for Lead.

42   Fiedorowicz, C. (n.d.). "Neurobiological Basis of Learning Disabilities." Retrieved February 04, 2008 from http://www. ldac-taac.ca/research/ neurobiological-e.asp.

43   Ibid.

44   US Department of Justice Office of Justice Programs Bureau of Justice Statistics. (1994). Violent Crime: National Crime Victimization Survey. Retrieved December 15, 2008 from http://www.ojp.usdoj.gov/bjs/pub/ascii/viocrm.txt.

45   Levitt, S.D. (2004). "Understanding why crime fell in the 1990s: four factors that explain the decline and six that do not." Journal of Economic Perspective, 18(1), 163-190.

46   Arizona School Association. "A Stranger Ignorance." Retrieved January 15, 2007 from http://www.azsba.org/lead3strange.htm.

47   Ibid.

48   Nevin, R. (2000). "How lead exposure relates to temporal changes in IQ, violent crime, and unwed pregnancy." Environmental Research Journal 83 (1), 1-22.

49   Ibid.

50   National Dairy Council. (2008). "Lactose Intolerance and Minorities: The Real Story." Retrieved September 28, 2008 from www.nationaldairycouncil.org.

51   Ibid.

52   Fulgoni, V., Nicholls, J., Reed, A., Buckley, R., DiRienzo, D., Miller, G.D. (2007). "Dairy consumption and related nutrient intake in African American adults and children in the United States: Continuing Survey of Food Intakes by Individuals 1994-1996 and the National Health and Nutrition Examination Survey 1999- 2000. "Journal of the American Dietetic Association. 107, 256-264.

53   Gentile, D.A., Lynch, P.J., Linder, J.R., & Walsh, D.A. (2004). "The effects of violent video game habits on adolescent hostility, aggressive behaviors, and school performance." Journal of Adolescence, 27, 5–22.

54   Reinberg, S. (2006). "Video game violence goes straight to kids' heads." Washington Post. Retrieved September 28, 2008 from www.washingtonpost.com.

55   Gurvits, T.V., Gilbertson, M.W., Lasko, N.B., Tarhan, A.S., Simeon, D., Macklin, M.L., Orr, S.P., & Pitman, R.K. (2000). "Neurologic soft signs in chronic posttraumatic stress disorder." Archives of General Psychiatry, 57, 181-186.

56   Ibid.

57   Tarter, R.E., Mezzich, A.C., Hsieh, Y.C., & Parks, S.M. (1995). "Cognitive capacity in female adolescent substance abusers." Drug and Alcohol Dependence, 39, 15-21.

58   Stocker, S. (1999). "Medications reduce incidence of substance abuse among ADHD patients." NIDA, 14, 6-8.

59   Needleman, H.L., McFarland, C., Ness, R.B., Feinberg, S.E., & Tobin, M.J. (2002). "Bone lead levels in adjudicated delinquents: a case control study." Neurotoxicology and Teratology, 24. 711-717.

60   Denno, D. (1990). Biology and Violence: From Birth to Adulthood. Cambridge University Press.

61   Dean, T.A. (2005). "A computational model of the cerebral cortex." Proceedings of Twentieth National Conference on Artificial Intelligence. Cambridge, Massachusetts: MIT Press, 938-943.

62 Needleman, H. L. (1993). "The current status of childhood low-level lead toxicity." Neurotoxicology, 14(2-3), 161-6.

63 Wilson, M.A., Johnston, M.V., Goldstein, G.W., & Blue, M.E. (2000). "Neonatal lead exposure impairs development of rodent barrel field cortex." PNAS, 97 (10), 5540-5545.

64 Needleman, H.L., McFarland, C., Ness, R.B., Feinberg, S.E., & Tobin, M.J. (2002). "Bone lead levels in adjudicated delinquents: A case control study." Neurotoxicology and Teratology, 24(6), 711-717.

65 Canfield, R.L., Henderson, C.R., Cory-Slechta, D.A., Cox, C., Jusko, T.A., & Lanphear, P.B. (2003). "Intellectual impairment in children with blood lead concentrations below 10 micrograms per deciliter." New England Journal of Medicine, 384, 1517-1526.

66 Salkever, D.S. (1995). "Updated estimates of earnings benefits from reduced exposure of children to environmental lead." Environmental Research 70, 1-6.

67 Sanghavi, D. "Getting the lead out." Slate Magazine. August 21, 2007.

68 Gordon, G.F. (2005). "Testosterone, a key to understanding mercury–autism link?" Autism Research Review, 19(1).

69 Geier, M.R., Geier, D.A. (2005). "The potential importance of steroids in the treatment of autistic spectrum disorders and other disorders involving mercury toxicity." Medical Hypotheses, 64(5), 946-54.

70 Autism Disability Data Source: The Individuals with Disabilities Education Act (IDEA) requires each state and the US Department of Education to record specific childhood disabilities including autism. This data was obtained from the US Department of Education at the www.ideadata.org.

71 Brock, S., Jimerson, S.R., & Hansen, R. (2006). Identifying, Assessing and Treating Autism at School. New York: Springer.

72 Accardo, P., Whitman, B., Caul, J., & Rolfe, U. (1988). "Autism and plumbism, a possible association." Clinical Pediatrics, 27(1), 41-44.

73 Cohen, D.J., Johnson, W.T., & Caparulo, B.K. (1976). "Pica and elevated blood lead level in autistic and atypical children." Archives of Pediatrics and Adolescent Medicine, 130(1).

74 Lidsky, T.I., & Schneider, J.S. (2005). "Autism and autistic symptoms associated with childhood lead poisoning." Journal of Applied Research, 5(1), 80-87.

75 Deisigner, J.A. (2001). Diagnosis and assessment of autistic spectrum disorders. In Wahlberg, T., Obiakor, F., Burkhardt, S., & Rotatori, A.F. (Eds.) "Autistic spectrum disorders: Educational and clinical interventions." Advances in Special Education, 14, 181-209.

76 Hoshino, Y., Kumashiro, H., Yashima, Y., Tachibana, R., & Watanabe, M. (1982). "The epidemiological study of autism in Fukushima-ken." Folia Psychiatry and Neurology Japan, 36, 115-124.

77 University of Wisconsin. "About mercury, another toxic metal." Retrieved November 14, 2007 from http://www.uwsp.edu/geo/courses/geog100/Lead- Mercury.htm.

78   Lotter, V. (1974). "Social adjustment and placement of autistic children in Middlesex: a follow-up study." Journal of Autism and Developmental Disorders, 4(1), 11-32.

79   Better Health Channel, "Pink Disease." Retrieved September 14, 2007 from http://www.betterhealth.vic.gov.au.

80   Stratton, K., Gable, A., & McCormick, M.C. (Eds.). (2001). Immunization Safety Review: Thimerosal–Containing Vaccines and Neurodevelopmental Disorders. Immunization Safety Review Committee, Board on Health Promotion and Disease Prevention.

81   Null, G. (2001). "Mercury Dental Amalgams: Analyzing the Debate." Retrieved September 25, 2007 from http://www.garynull.com/documents/Dental/ Amalgam/Amalgam2.htm.

82   Talbot, E.S. (1883). "Injurious effects of mercury as used in dentistry." Missouri Dentistry Journal, 15, 124-30.

83   International Medical Veritas Association." Disease Forming Toxic Waste Dumps." Retrieved November 23, 2007 from http://www.imva.info/vaporsfromhell.shtml.

84   Talbot, E.S. (1883). "Injurious effects of mercury as used in dentistry." Missouri Dentistry Journal, 15, 124-30.

85   Null, G. (2001). "Mercury Dental Amalgams: Analyzing the Debate." Retrieved September 25, 2007 from http://www.garynull.com/documents/Dental/ Amalgam/Amalgam2.htm.

86   DAMS Inc. (2005). Mercury Free and Healthy. Saint Paul: MN.

87   Null, G. (2001). "Mercury Dental Amalgams: Analyzing the Debate." Retrieved September 25, 2007 from http://www.garynull.com/documents/Dental/ Amalgam/Amalgam2.htm.

88   Environment Canada. "Mercury and the Environment."
      Retrieved July 05, 2008 from http://www.ec.gc.ca/MERCURY/
      EN/index.cfm.

89   The Canadian Council of Ministers of the Environment.
      "Canada-Wide Standard on Mercury for Dental Amalgam
      Waste." Retrieved July 13, 2008 from http://www.ccme.ca/
      assets/pdf/cws_merc_amalgam_e.pdf.

90   Huggins, H.A. Monographs on Mercury. Huggins
      Applied Healing. Retrieved February 26, 2007 from
      http://www.hugginsappliedhealing.com/store/product.
      php?productid=16163.

91   Bernard, S., Enayati, A., Redwood, L., Roger, H., & Binstock,
      T. (2001)." Autism: a novel type of mercury poisoning."
      Medical Hypothesis 56(4), 462-471.

92   Dador, D.E. (2007). "Lead poisoning often confused for
      autism." Healthy Living. Retrieved September 25, 2008
      from http://abclocal.go.com/kabc/ story?section=news/
      health&id=5828838.

93   Kennedy, R. (2005). "Deadly Immunity." Retrieved December
      12, 2007 from http://www.commondreams.org/views05/0616-
      31.htm.

94   Olmsted, D. (2007). "The Age of Autism: The Last Word."
      Retrieved April 24, 2008 from http://www.whale.to/vaccine/
      olmsted.html.

95   Wedeen, R.P. (1984). Poison in the Pot. The Legacy of
      Lead. Southern Illinois University Press, Carbondale and
      Edwardsville.

96   Bell, J.U., & Thomas, J.A. (1980). "Effects of Lead in Mammalian Reproduction. " In Lead Toxicity R. L. Singhal and J.A. Thomas, (Eds.), Baltimore-Munich: Urban and Schwarzenberg.

97   Bhattacharya, S. "Lead may cause mystery male infertility." New Scientist. February 06, 2003.

98   Needleman, H.L., & Landrigan, P.J. (1994). Raising Children Toxic Free. New York: Farrar, Straus and Giroux.

99   Pergament, E., Schechtman, A., & Koval, C. (1995). "Lead exposure in pregnancy." Risk Newsletter. Illinois Department of Public Health. Retrieved July 28, 2008 from http://www.fetal-exposure.org/LEAD.html.

100 West, W.L., Knight, E.M., Edwards, C.H., Manning, M., Spurlock, B., James, H., Johnson, A.A., Oyemade, U.J., Cole, O.J., Westney, O.E., Laryea, H., Jones, S., & Westney, L. S. (1994). "Maternal low level lead and pregnancy outcomes." Journal of Nutrition, 124 (6), 981-986.

101 National Academy of Sciences. (1993). Pesticides in the Diets of Infants and Children. National Academy Press. Washington, DC.

102 Environmental Working Group. (2005). Body Burden: The Pollution in Newborns. Washington, D.C.

103 Needleman, H.L., & Landrigan, P.J. (1994). Raising Children Toxic Free. New York: Farrar, Straus and Giroux

104 Alternative Doctor. "Heavy Metal Poisoning." Retrieved December 14, 2007 from http://www.alternative-doctor.com/anti-ageing/heavy_metal.html.

105 Schettler, T., Stein, J., Reich, F., Valenti, M., & Wallinga, D. (2000). In Harm's Way. Greater Boston Physicians for Social Responsibility.

106 Ibid.

107 Bonithon-Kopp, C., Huel, G., Moreau, T., Wendling, R. (1986). "Prenatal exposure to lead and cadmium and psychomotor development of the child at 6 years." Neurobehavioral Toxicology and Teratology 8(3), 307-310.

108 Alternative Doctor. "Heavy Metal Poisoning." Retrieved December 14, 2007 from http://www.alternative-doctor.com/anti-ageing/heavy_metal.html.

109 Tjalve, H., Henriksson, J., & Tallkvist, J. (1996). "Uptake of manganese and cadmium from the nasal mucosa into the central nervous system via olfactory pathways in rats." Pharmacology and Toxicology, 79, 347-356.

110 Schettler, T., Stein, J., Reich, F., Valenti, M., & Wallinga, D. (2000). In Harm's Way. Greater Boston Physicians for Social Responsibility.

111 Ibid.

112 Ibid.

113 Bisphenol A. "About Bisphenol A." Retrieved February 14, 2008 from http://www.bisphenol-a.org/about/index.html.

114 Calafat, A.M., Kuklenyik, Z., Reidy, J.A., Claudill, S.P., Ekong, J., & Needham. H.L. (2005)." Urinary concentrations of Bisphenol A and 4-Nonylphenol in a human reference population." Environmental Health Perspectives, 113(4), 391-395.

115   Dioxin Homepage. Retrieved January 20, 2008, from: http://www.ejnet.org/dioxin/.

116   Ibid.

117   Gibbs, L.M. (1982). Love canal: My story. Albany, State University of New York Press.

118   US Food and Drug Administration (2006). "Questions and Answers about Dioxins." Retrieved February 14, 2008 from http://vm.cfsan.fda.gov/~lrd/dioxinqa.html.

119   Washington State Department of Ecology. "PBDE Flame Retardants: A Fast-growing Concern." Retrieved February 7, 2008, from: http://www.ecy.wa.gov/programs/eap/pbt/pbde/.

120   Needleman, H.L., & Landrigan, P.J. (1994). Raising Children Toxic Free. New York: Farrar, Straus and Giroux.

121   The Canadian Association of Physicians for the Environment. Retrieved January 20, 2008 from http://www.cape.ca/children/neuro5.html.

122   Environmental Protection Agency. "Health Effects of PCBs." Retrieved January 14, 2008 from http://www.epa.gov.

123   Chen, Y.C., Guo, Y.L. Hsu, C.C., & Rogan, W.J. (1992). "Cognitive development of Yu-Cheng ("oil disease") children prenatally exposed to heat-degraded PCBs." Journal of American Medical Association, 268(22), 3213-3218.

124   Schettler, T., Stein, J., Reich, F., Valenti, M., & Wallinga, D. (2000). In Harm's Way. Greater Boston Physicians for Social Responsibility.

125 The Canadian Association of Physicians for the Environment. Retrieved January 20, 2008 from http://www.cape.ca/toxics/pesticides.html.

126 Centers for Disease Control and Prevention. (2005). Third National Report on Human Exposure to Environmental Chemicals. Atlanta (GA): CDC.

127 Environmental Working Group. (2005). Body Burden: The Pollution in Newborns. Washington, D.C.

128 Canadian Association of Physicians for the Environment. "Pesticides." Retrieved January 24, 2008 from www.cape.ca/children/neuro6html.

129 Schettler, T., Stein, J., Reich, F., Valenti, M., & Wallinga, D. (2000). In Harm's Way. Greater Boston Physicians for Social Responsibility.

130 Colborn, T., Dumanoski, D., & Myers, J.P. (1996). Our Stolen Future. New York: Dutton.

131 UK Ministry of Agriculture, Fisheries and Food. (1996). "Phthalates in Infant Formulae." Retrieved April 28, 2008 from http://www.infactcanada.ca/phthalat.htm.

132 UK Ministry of Agriculture, Fisheries and Food. (1996). "Phthalates in Food." Retrieved from http://website.lineone.net/~mwarhurst/phthalates.html.

133 Jobling, S., Reynolds, T., White, R., Parker, M.G. & Sumpter, J.P. (1995)." A variety of environmentally persistent chemicals, including some phthalate plasticizers, are weakly estrogenic." Environmental Health Perspectives, 103, 582-587.

134 Sathynarayana, S., Karr, C.J., Lozano, P., Brown, E., Calafat, A.M., Fan Liu, & Swan, S.H. (2008). "Baby care products: possible sources of infant phthalate exposure." Pediatrics, 121, e260-e268.

135 Committee on the Environment Public Health and Food Safety. "Phthalates in toys and child care articles." Retrieved December 30, 2007 from www.europarl.europa.eu/.

136 Volk, B., Maletz, M., Tiedemann, M., Mall, G., Klein, C., & Berlet, H.H. (1981). "Impaired maturation of Purkinje cells in the fetal alcohol syndrome of the rat." Acta Neuropathologica, 54(1), 19-29.

137 Hernandez-Avila, M., Gonzalez-Cossio, T., Hernandez-Avila, J.E., Romier, I., Peterson, K.E., Aro, A., Palazuelos, E., Kageyama Escobar, M.L., & Hu, H. (2003). "Dietary calcium supplements to lower blood lead levels in lactating women: a randomized placebo-controlled trial." Epidemiology, 14(2), 206-12.

138 Simon, J.A., & Hudes, E.S. (1999). "Relationship of ascorbic acid to blood lead levels." Journal of the American Medical Association, 281(24), 228-229

139 Aga, M., Iwaki, K., Ueda, Y., Shipmpei, U., Masaki, N., Fukuda, S., Kimoto, T., Ikeda, M., & Kurimoto, M. (2001)." Preventative effect of Coriandrum sativum (Chinese parsley) on localized lead deposition in ICR mice." Journal of Ethnopharmacology, 77, (2-3): 203-8.

140 Omura, Y., Shimotsuura, Y., Fukuoka, A., Fukuoka, H., & Nomoto, T. (1996). "Significant mercury deposits in internal organs following the removal of dental amalgam, & development of pre-cancer on the gingiva and the sides of the tongue and their represented organs as a result of inadvertent exposure to strong curing light (used to solidify synthetic dental filling material) & effective treatment: a clinical case report, along with organ representation areas for each tooth." Acupuncture Electrotherapy Research, 21(2), 133-160.

141 Wellness Directory of Minnesota. (n.d.) "Cilantro: A Common Spice/Herb That Can Save Your Life." Retrieved April 24, 2008 from www.mnwelldir.org/docs/ cilantro.htm.

142 Queiroz, M., Torello, C.O., Perhs, S.M. et al. (2008). "Chlorella vulgaris up- modulation of myelossupression induced by lead: the role of stromal cells." Food and Chemical Toxicology, 46(9), 3147-3154.

143 Dolby, V. (1995) "Garlic comes through with another benefit: detoxifying the body." Better Nutrition. (August).